THE

REFERENCE

SHELF

THE CRISIS IN
HEALTH CARE

edited by ROBERT EMMET LONG

THE REFERENCE SHELF

Volume 63 Number 1

*RA
395
·A3
C83
1991*

THE H. W. WILSON COMPANY

New York   1991

THE REFERENCE SHELF

The books in this series contain reprints of articles, excerpts from books, and addresses on current issues and social trends in the United States and other countries. There are six separately bound numbers in each volume, all of which are generally published in the same calendar year. One number is a collection of recent speeches; each of the others is devoted to a single subject and gives background information and discussion from various points of view, concluding with a comprehensive bibliography that contains books and pamphlets and abstracts of additional articles on the subject. Books in the series may be purchased individually or on subscription.

Library of Congress Cataloging-in-Publication Data

Main entry under title:

Printed in the United States of America

CONTENTS

Health care in America has become a source of concern as perhaps never before. The last decade in particular has witnessed an unprecedented escalation of costs for medical treatment and for the health insurance with which to defray it. Treatment of a fractured ankle may sometimes cost thousands of dollars, a staggering sum yet small compared to the astronomical cost of major surgery, a protracted stay in a hospital, or living in a nursing home. The first of the four sections of this collection raises the question of how and why health care costs have reached such disturbing levels, and what is being done or can be done to contain them. Ironically, the beginning of the upward spiral resulted from a humanitarian effort to provide greater health protection for a larger number of Americans. The passage of Medicare and Medicaid in the mid-1960s, part of Lyndon Johnson's Great Society legislation, increased health care coverage but, since the government would be writing the checks, provided no incentive for doctors or hospitals to limit their fees. In the same period extraordinary advances occurred in medical science and technology, opening a large new field of ultra-expensive medical care treatment. As ailing Americans began to demand the best care available, even if obtained at enormously expensive cost, an enormous new health care industry has come into being, and raising questions of many kinds. Most of all, it raises the question of equity and fairness, as the affluent, the not-so-well-off, and the poor have vastly different access to the health care community.

The second section examines the situation of health care providers. Doctors today belong to a large medical establishment, frequently serving giant hospital complexes or other medical corporations called health maintenance organizations (HMOs). Regulations are set by management executives and cost accountants. This depersonalization of medical care tends to create an atmosphere of mutual distrust between patient and physician. Citizens wonder anxiously if they can afford to become ill, while doctors are ever conscious that they may be subjected to the vastly increasing number of malpractice suits. The economics of the new medical care is a factor, particularly in the inception and vast expansion of for-profit hospital chains that cater to the well-to-do, while the poor or those with inadequate insurance or none at all are relegated to public hospitals with deteriorating facilities, whose staffs are overworked and whose budgets are constrained or uncertain. This situation resembles the flight of the affluent to the suburbs while the needy inhabit the deteriorating inner cities. Medicine is tiered according to class.

The third section addresses the situation of the elderly, whose numbers are continually increasing because of medical breakthroughs and advances in technology. The so-called graying of America places special stresses on the management and financing of the medical care economy and raises troubling questions about the rationing of health services. Ethicists in medicine wonder whether it will be possible to provide expensive treatment to the elderly without creating an unacceptable burden on younger taxpayers. At the same time, older citizens feel anxiety about coping with the runaway cost of health care that comes when illness and incapacity strike. Nursing home confinement is so expensive that individuals' lifetime savings are quickly depleted.

In the final section, writers from the medical, corporate, and political communities debate the desirability of a national health care system. Although controversial, a national health insurance plan of some kind is now advocated by many different groups. Large corporations until now provided a large share of health insurance costs for their workers and retirees, but such expenditures have grown so large and cut so heavily into profit margins that corporate executives have cut back on health care contributions—and even advocate a government-funded health care system. Union leaders and members of congress, among others, have advanced proposals for such a system, some pointing to the Canadian health care system as a prospective model. As the concluding articles in this section indicate, however, the Canadian system is flawed in many respects and would not seem hospitable to the individualistic ethos and consumer demands of Americans.

The editor is indebted to the authors and publishers who have granted permission to reprint the materials in this compilation. Special thanks are due to Joyce Cook and the Fulton (N.Y.) Public Library staff, to Fulton's G. Ray Bodley school library, and to the staff of Penfield Library, State University of New York at Oswego.

ROBERT EMMET LONG

November 1990

I. THE SOARING COST OF HEALTH CARE

EDITOR'S INTRODUCTION

Throughout the 1980s the cost of health care in the United States has been rising steadily and steeply, becoming a matter of concern to everyone. The spector facing the elderly is that they may be unable to meet medical costs at a time when they are most in need of medical treatment. The cost of nursing home care now ranges between $25,000 and $50,000 annually, a figure that quickly deprives the aged of the security they felt they had. Once their savings are gone, they may still have nursing home care, but they will, in effect, be wards of the state, reduced to pauperdom. Those of all ages feel anxiety as the expense of medical treatment escalates. Millions of Americans have no health insurance at all, and are thus in a helpless position when an injury or serious health problem strikes. The wealthy may be shielded by their personal resources from the calamity of catastrophic illness, but all others—the bulk of the population—are at risk. Chapter One of this collection focuses upon the runaway cost of medical care, its causes and consequences.

In the first article, reprinted from the *New York Times Magazine,* Joseph Califano, former Secretary of Health, Education, and Welfare, traces the dilemma of spiralling health costs to the establishment of the Medicare and Medicaid programs in the mid 1960s, which were designed to provide security for large numbers of Americans. The programs, however, offered no incentive for providers of health care to keep costs down. Even when it was recognized that abuses were occurring, nothing was done to reform the programs because powerful interests were involved. Health care, as Califano points out, is one of America's three largest industries, with tremendous influence on political decision-making in Washington. Califano points particularly to the increased use of extremely expensive surgical procedures, used either inappropriately or with uncertain value to patients.

In the next article, from *The New Leader,* George P. Brockway discusses efforts to cope with the problem of health insurance, pointing particularly to the Massachusetts plan, which requires all employers to insure their employees, while the state insures the balance of the uninsured population. But, as Brockway points out, if unemployment in the state became high, the burden on the state budget would become severe. Moreover, small or marginal businesses would be especially hard hit by the costs of insuring their employees, and business generally would be reluctant to hire new people and thus increase their insurance burden. Next, in an article reprinted from *Consumer's Research Magazine,* Gregory Hoelscher and Carolyn Lochhead look at a variety of attempts to contain medical care expenses. The federal government, for example, has imposed on hospitals a fee reimbursement schedule for 468 categories of illness, called Diagnostic-Related Groups, or DRGs. Hospitals charging more than the DRG rates must assume the additional cost themselves. Health Maintenance Organizations, or HMOs, are also favored by insurance-carrying employers, since HMOs charge a company a fixed annual fee for all medical services, reducing the incentive to build up costs. Finally, writing in *USA Today,* Donald G. Lightfoot discusses the increasing awareness of employers that they need to educate their workers in good health practices and to initiate company exercise programs—both of which have reduced health insurance claims.

THE HEALTH-CARE CHAOS[1]

Just as history teaches that war is too important to be left to generals, so recent American experience teaches that medicine is too important to be left to doctors and politicians.

Health is devouring an ever-increasing share of our national wealth: Americans will spend more than $550 billion on health care this year; that's nearing 12 percent of our gross national product. For years, Medicare has been the fastest growing part of our Federal budget. And it's becoming increasingly clear that a large portion of the money spent on health care is wasted.

Congress over the years has contributed at least as much to

[1]Reprint of a magazine article by Joseph Califano, former Secretary of Health, Education and Welfare (1977–1979). From the *New York Times Magazine,* Nov 20 '88. pg. 44, 46, 56–58. Copyright © 1988 by the New York Times Company. Reprinted by Permission.

the problem as to the solution. Take the catastrophic-care bills now before a House and Senate conference committee. Surely Americans should be protected from the financial ruin that catastrophic illness can bring—but efficiently. These bills offer few incentives to physicians and patients to choose less expensive alternatives to hospital care, and even fewer measures to control other costs. As drafted, the legislation represents a reckless insistence that the last quarter century has nothing to teach: it is likely to spark a surge of spending on high-ticket, high-tech medicine, setting us back years in our cost-containment efforts. It will surely cost far more than Congress estimates, maybe twice as much. [The Medicare Catastrophic Coverage Act was passed by Congress in 1988, then repealed in 1989 after public outcry against it as a tax increase.]

To understand why Congress is likely to pass legislation that will once again open the taxpayers' checkbooks to the doctors and hospitals, lining the pockets of health-care providers under cover of caring for patients, one has to look a little more closely at the politics of health care.

For example, both the House and Senate bills provide a new prescription-drug benefit—which is fine, indeed vital. But though the Government would pick up the tab for the patient's pharmaceuticals, it would also pay a fee to the pharmacy or to the mail-order supplier of $4.50 a prescription—even though it is estimated that a mail-order supplier charges its corporate health-plan clients only 50 cents to fill a prescription and process a claim.

The most energetic lobby behind the new drug benefit is the American Association of Retired Persons, which runs the country's second-largest mail-order drug-dispensing business (1986 revenues: $200 million). That $4.50 dispensing fee represents a substantial windfall for the politically powerful A.A.R.P.

Domination of the political process by health-care providers is not new. In 1964, when President Lyndon B. Johnson proposed the Medicare and Medicaid programs, Congress demanded as the price of passage that the programs stipulate "cost-plus" reimbursement for hospitals and the prevailing "fee-for-service" payments for doctors.

In 1968, Johnson urged that these systems be reformed, arguing that they offered doctors no incentive to provide care efficiently. Johnson's warning that without a change in reimbursement costs would reach $100 billion by 1975 was ridiculed on Capitol Hill. In fact, that year costs exceeded $130 billion.

Every President since has sought to limit increases in health-care costs. Congress after Congress has rebuffed them. (Congress has repeatedly increased payments to hospitals beyond the Reagan Administration's recommendations—adding at least $500 million a year to the budget—even though American hospitals have some 400,000 empty beds, a huge excess capacity they refuse to reduce.)

During the two years leading up to the 1986 elections, those in the health-care industry channeled more than $8.5 million through various political action committees to members of Congress. Next to financial services, this is more than any other industry—more than the handgun and tobacco lobbies, the oil companies and the 100 largest defense contractors. And that $8.5 million does not include direct contributions made by doctors and hospital administrators. For the contributors, those political gifts are a small price to pay to keep a piece of one of America's three largest industries.

Dramatic, convulsive change marks the business of American health care. Miracle drugs are eliminating childhood diseases, tempering depression, taming epilepsy, and so revolutionizing the treatment of coronary disease that heart surgeons may soon find their specialty as obsolete as picking cotton by hand. And just over the horizon lies a barely explored world of biotechnology beyond the imagination of Steven Spielberg.

Yet the more turmoil and change there is, the more one thing remains the same: health-care costs keep skyrocketing. During 1986 and 1987 the price of American health care shot up at more than twice the rate of inflation. The rise in physicians' fees and services was so steep last year that Medicare had to increase the premiums people pay for physician care by nearly 40 percent. Health-insurance premiums are up an average of almost 20 percent this year, with some increases a dizzying 70 percent.

The evidence is growing that at least a quarter of this money—more than $125 billion—will be wasted; $25 billion of that comes from the taxpayer. At a time when Congress is agonizing over budget cuts of less than that amount, when 37 million Americans are going without even basic health insurance, and when American companies are struggling to cut costs to meet foreign competition, such waste is unconscionable.

So far, government, big business, and unions—the main providers of health care—have primarily used blunt instruments to hack fat out of the bloated health-care system. They have concentrated on creating incentives for doctors and patients to eliminate unnecessary hospital stays and shorten necessary ones, and they've had some success.

But now comes the tough part: finding out what treatments really work; instilling self-discipline in patients, physicians and politicians; and directing Americans' scientific genius toward the health-care problems that actually cost Americans the most money—and the most misery.

Of the tasks ahead, none is more complex than finding out what procedures truly have an impact on the ailment the patient suffers—in short, determining what quality care really is. Americans spent almost $1,800 a person on health care in 1985—far more than the Canadians, who ranked second ($1,300), more than twice the Japanese ($800), and triple the British ($600). Yet health care in Canada, Japan and Britain is sophisticated and modern, life expectancy is at least as high as in the United States, and infant mortality is lower.

We are so dazzled by the miracles of modern medicine we tend to forget that even today, despite the multimillion-dollar array of tools at the doctor's disposal, the first step—correctly diagnosing the ailment—is no sure bet. And treatments for the same diagnosis vary widely.

In 1987, a pioneering researcher named Dr. John E. Wennberg compared surgery and hospitalization rates in New Haven and Boston. He found that, in 1982, a New Haven resident was nearly twice as likely to undergo a coronary bypass operation as a Bostonian, but only half as likely to receive a carotid endarterectomy. Bostonians were much more likely to have their knees and hips replaced, but New Haven residents had far more hysterectomies and back operations. Boston doctors will hospitalize you for gastroenteritis, pneumonia and diabetes much more readily than their colleagues in New Haven.

These different treatments, applied to populations that are essentially very similar, appeared to bear *no relation* to whether the patients gets well. But they did bear a strong relation to the cost: Medicare spent an average of 70 percent more for each beneficiary in Boston than it did in New Haven. That's a heavy price to pay—especially when the Bostonian's chance of being exposed to a more expensive, higher-risk procedure appears to depend not on his condition, but on the prevailing fashion in his medical neighborhood.

Another study, this one by the Rand Corporation, analyzing

4.4 million Medicare beneficiaries, revealed wide variations in rates for surgery and hospitalization. Consider two patients, one of whom happens to live in the area that had the highest rate for a particular procedure, the other in the area with the lowest rate. The first patient was 11 times more likely to have a hip operation, 6 times more likely to have a knee replaced, 3 times more likely to have coronary bypass surgery, 5 times more likely to have a skin biopsy. For more than half of the medical and surgical procedures studied (67 out of 123), people who lived in areas with the highest rate were at least three times as likely to undergo the procedure as people living in areas with the lowest rate.

In a subsequent Rand study, medical experts meticulously analyzed the application of three of the procedures, first reviewing the research on its effectiveness and establishing criteria for when it was clearly appropriate, clearly inappropriate, or of uncertain value. After systematically applying these criteria to 4,564 case histories, the experts found that 26 percent of coronary angiographies (a procedure to determine blockage of coronary arteries); 28 percent of endoscopies (a procedure to diagnose stomach and intestinal problems), and 64 percent of carotid endarterectomies (a surgical procedure to remove blockages from the main artery supplying blood to the brain) were clearly inappropriate or of uncertain value. Most startling, researchers found that when they compared communities with the highest and lowest rates, the rate of inappropriate use was about the same.

So we have an expert medical consensus that from 26 to 64 percent of these three medical procedures were of no value or of uncertain value to the patients. But even when most doctors agree that certain treatments *are* appropriate, there are still enormous variations—some more than tenfold—in the rates at which people living in different places are subjected to risky, expensive surgical procedures—with no apparent relation to their health.

What accounts for these stunning variations in treatment? Probably not differences in medical training: there are fewer than 130 medical schools in the United States, and their curriculums have been pretty much standardized for 50 years. And the incidence of common ailments does not appear to fluctuate significantly from region to region.

Is it possible that in this era of high-tech medicine we just don't know with any precision whether many procedures truly affect the medical outcome? Certainly it is.

But there are situations in which we should be able to develop standards of care and apply them, situations in which doctors clearly are too ready to choose surgery:

• Coronary bypasses. Americans are four times more likely to have bypass operations than Western Europeans with the same symptoms. According to studies by the National Institutes of Health and the Veterans Administration, at least 60 percent, and perhaps 80 percent, of the 250,000 Americans who undergo coronary bypass surgery each year gain no increase in life span beyond what they would have achieved through medical management of their conditions. Henry J. Aaron and Dr. William B. Schwartz, in their book "The Painful Prescription," attribute much of the rapid growth in the use of bypass surgery to the fee-for-service payment system (coronary bypasses cost about $25,000 each).

• Caesarean sections. In 1970, 5.5 percent of the deliveries of babies in the United States were Caesarean; in 1986, 24 percent were. Medical experts estimate that at least half of the 900,000 C-sections performed in 1986 were unnecessary. The cost of those excess operations came to $728 million—for poor quality medicine. American doctors perform the highest rate of Caesarean sections in the world, yet the United States ranks 17th in infant mortality.

• Tonsillectomies. If you want to keep your tonsils, stay out of Fairhaven, Fitchburg and Framingham, Mass. Residents of these cities were found to be as much as 15 times more likely to be subjected to tonsillectomies than residents of other Bay State towns, where tonsillitis is treated mainly with antibiotics—as effectively, and more cheaply.

• Pacemaker Implants. Recent studies suggest that of the 120,000 pacemaker implants performed annually—at a cost of $1.5 billion—more than half are unnecessary or of questionable value. A Philadelphia study suggested that doctors' ignorance and the fear of malpractice accusations were the chief culprits; but the study also noted that this relatively simple operation, with its $12,000 price tag, can be highly profitable for doctors and hospitals.

I'm not suggesting that all the varying judgments of doctors on what constitutes appropriate care are unreasonable, reckless, or motivated by economic self-interest. In many cases, one physician may in good conscience perform surgery though another may treat the same condition medically.

I do suggest that a major shift in physician and patient attitudes would improve the quality of care. Right now, when a physician is uncertain about the value of a medical procedure, his attitude tends to be: unless it has been proved ineffective, try it. Patients in discomfort tend to agree. In a medical system in which doctors are paid only for doing *something,* and patients want something done, uncertainty over diagnosis and treatment makes for all kinds of unnecessary tests and treatments.

I suggest we adopt a different attitude: unless the procedure has been proved effective, don't use it. There is ample precedent for this. After all, drug companies routinely spend millions of dollars demonstrating the safety and effectiveness of their products, in order to convince the Food and Drug Administration to let them bring new drugs to market. Yet most medical and surgical procedures—which are far more costly and risky—are subjected to far less scrutiny before they are adopted.

It's time for a rigorous effort to establish what procedures produce beneficial outcomes under what conditions—and to eliminate stark instances of "overutilization" like those cited above. Physicians and hospital administrators should put establishing quality standards at the top of their agendas.

If the professionals procrastinate, government and other big buyers of health care will act. Surging costs will spur these purchasers to insist that they will pay only for procedures that can be shown to affect the medical outcome. And, costs aside, subjecting patients to high-risk surgical procedures that have little or no likelihood of affecting their health raises profound ethical questions.

Defining quality health care will not be easy. We are trying to determine the best way to treat a patient, to judge the competence of doctors, nurses and lab technicians, and to quantify some intangibles. But computers make it simple to measure outcomes of medical procedures by analyzing rates of relapse, readmission, surgical rupture, infection, length of hospital stays, length of recovery time, time away from work, death rates and other data.

The Joint Commission on Accreditation of Health Care Organizations is in the midst of developing specific performance indicators. The United States Department of Health and Human Services has begun to publish the death rates of various hospitals, and to test quality standards for hospital intensive-care units. On the state level, the Pennsylvania legislature has created a Health Care Cost Containment Council to collect and publish data, gathered from every Pennsylvania physician and hospital, on what surgical and medical procedures are performed for what diagnoses, and on rates of infection, hospital readmission and mortality.

At the Chrysler Corporation, where I am chairman of the health-care committee of the board of directors, we are trying to set quality and cost-effective standards for our disability programs. A searching examination of our disability system revealed that 5 percent of the claims generated 40 percent of the costs; that employees holding the same job took widely varying leaves for the same ailments or injuries; and that, for certain procedures—appendectomies, cataract surgery, tonsillectomies and breast biopsies—hourly employees spent twice as many days on disability leave as expected, and many more than salaried employees.

Drawing on the expertise of 47 physicians, Chrysler established treatment options, which vary according to the employee's physical condition, job, age and sex, and then created guidelines for the appropriate length of disability leave.

During its first six months, Chrysler's program has saved more than $3 million, and 52,000 days of work. Physicians appreciate having standards that help them judge the length of disability, and resist patient pressure for more time off. Employees appreciate that objective standards are now applied fairly to everyone—and they undergo fewer questionable medical procedures.

Before we can persuade doctors to adopt standards of quality care, we must slay the medical-malpractice monster. Medical professionals should be held accountable for negligence and incompetence, but not for disappointment and grief over events no one can predict or control. States should follow California's lead by limiting recovery for damages to modest payment for pain and suffering, the cost of care, income lost because of missed work, and compensation for lingering disability. Contingent legal fees should be sharply reduced.

Physicians and hospitals should do their part by screening out doctors who provide substandard care. In 23 states the peer-review organizations of physicians set up by Congress to assure quality care have not imposed a single sanction.

We must pursue quality care without imposing "cookie-cutter medicine" and stifling the creativity that has made American medicine the envy of the world. But in areas in which standards can be established, they can serve as a safe haven for doctors, protecting them from unjustified malpractice claims.

We also need to bring about a major change in patients' attitudes. First, patients must recognize their responsibility to take care of themselves. We've lost sight of the only sure way to contain health-care costs: keeping people out of the sick-care system.

Of the $550 billion Americans spend on health care, less than 0.3 percent is spent on health promotion and disease prevention. Government, employers, schools, doctors and other health professionals—all have an interest in marketing health promotion with the same sophisticated saturation the ad agencies employ to sell products. The priorities are clear: quitting smoking, sticking to a proper diet, controlling drinking, taking regular exercise, learning to handle stress, practicing preventive care and having regular check-ups.

Patients have come to judge physicians by how much doctors do to them—how spectacular their diagnostic and treatment procedures are, how high-tech their offices and hospitals are. We must re-educate patients, promoting a cultural shift in patient attitudes. One way to begin is to pay doctors to *talk* to their patients, and to persuade patients that fees for that service are often better spent than those paying only for doctors to "do something" to them.

This shift in attitude must be achieved in the face of convictions that "nothing's too good or expensive for my sick baby"—or spouse, or parent. It must be achieved among a generation of Americans who pop tranquilizers not to relieve unusual stress but to subject themselves to even more; who rely on pills rather than self-discipline to avoid obesity, to relax, to sleep.

Finally, we must dramatically reorder our research priorities. In particular, we must direct money for medical research to our two largest problems: aging and addiction.

As people live longer, the length of time during which they need help in the tasks of daily living increases. The astronomical cost of confronting this dependence has sent tremors through Congress and state capitols, and has drained the savings and psyches of far more American families than catastrophic illness.

Millions of the elderly living at home need help with the basic activities of living. And of America's 1.3 million residents of nursing homes, 91 percent need help bathing; 77 percent need help dressing; 63 percent need help using the toilet; and more than 40 percent need help eating. Sixty-three percent suffer from dementia, mental disorientation, loss of memory.

We need a massive effort—a Project Independence for Older Americans—to reduce and, for many of the elderly, eliminate the chief threats to their independence. A Project Independence research program should focus on at least three areas; incontinence, memory loss and immobility.

Incontinence among the elderly is, as a *New England Journal of Medicine* article puts it, "prevalent, morbid, costly and neglected." Last year, more than $8 billion was spent to care for 500,000 incontinent elderly people in nursing homes. Yet even among the neglected area of research for the elderly, incontinence has been especially shunned.

Severe dementia afflicts some 1.5 million Americans so seriously that they require constant care; perhaps 5 million others suffer from mild to moderate dementia. Americans spend $40 billion to $50 billion a year to care for elderly dementia victims, yet last year we spent less than $80 million on research on all forms of elderly dementia.

Almost 2 million Americans over 65 need help just walking across a room. Ninety percent of all women over 75 suffer from osteoporosis. Arthritis afflicts some 15 million elderly Americans, at a cost exceeding $3.5 billion last year; yet we invested only $138 million in research on arthritis.

The more independent the elderly are, the less expensive nursing and institutional care they require. Independence is what the elderly want most. Is there any son or daughter who would rather spend money to keep parents in a nursing home than to keep them living independently? The payoff of Project Independence for Older Americans could be enormous. Each reduction of one month in the average period of dependence means a savings of up to $4 billion in health care and custodial costs.

We must also reorient our research efforts toward addiction. The cost of addiction in health care alone easily exceeds $50 billion. Yet out of a total research budget of $6 billion, the Government spends less than $200 million to learn about addiction. And alcoholism, despite the widespread diseases it causes, is near the bottom of the list in private research support.

Fifty-four million Americans are addicted to cigarettes; 18 million are addicted to or abuse alcohol; half a million, heroin; at least ten million abuse barbiturates and other sedative-hypnotic drugs. Sixty million Americans have used marijuana; up to 22 million have tried cocaine—no one knows exactly how many of them are dependent, in one way or another, on those drugs.

If we're serious about reducing the demand for drugs, we must begin by finding out why people become addicted. Yet it has been difficult to get our best scientific minds concentrated on addiction—in part because the problem is so infernally complex, and in part because the financing has been erratic. The United States should establish a national institute of addiction, as part of the National Institutes of Health, which would combine the research work of the National Institute on Drug Abuse and on Alcohol Abuse and Alcoholism. This institute would conduct research on all substance abuse, including smoking. By creating a single institute for all addiction research, Congress would help generate a steady stream of money, make clear our national commitment and attract more of our best minds to the effort.

Picture our health-care system as a mountain-climbing team struggling to scale an extremely steep cliff en route to a Mount Everest of quality care for all.

The lead climber is our spectacular scientific genius and superb doctors and medical centers. But then come those who have lost their footing. One dangling climber is the hospitals, with their empty beds. Another is technology, swinging loose on the rope, unbridled by considerations of the relationship of cost to benefit. Next come lawyers and judges, dragging the team down with malpractice litigation. Then the enormous load of patient expectations, crying out: Do something, Doctor, up to the limit of my health insurance—and don't hold me responsible for my own health. Finally, comes the politician, pandering to providers, needlessly adding to the cost of care.

Our lead climber must negotiate this slippery cliff in a blinding snowstorm of uncertainty about which medical and surgical procedures truly affect the medical outcome for patients. In a sense, it's remarkable that our health-care system is still scaling the cliff. But it cannot hope to reach the heights of quality care for all unless we get all members of the team to do their share. Bluntly put, we are talking about the continued viability of America's top-quality medical system.

Whether we maintain and enhance that system—and make it available to all our citizens—is not a decision to be left in the hands of physicians and politicians. It is a decision for all of us—employers and unions, patients and citizens.

MEDICAL CARE AND PAUPERIZATION[2]

Having recently seen the insides of more hospitals than I wanted, and having accordingly had bills from more medical specialists than I dreamed existed, I have a more intimate awareness of the Medigap than I had when I wrote . . . [previously] on the subject. Hence these reflections on three related problems.

First, I have an unhappy impression that some of the specialists were unnecessary, and that some of the things the necessary ones charged for were unnecessary. A couple seemed to drop around for two or three minutes of bedside chit-chat long after the diagnosis had been made and their specialty's noninvolvement confirmed.

One of the latter, a nice fellow with an impressive beard, sent me a bill for 12 such visits at $65 a pop. Medicare will ultimately pay somewhat less than one-half of that, and a group policy I have will probably pick up 80 per cent of the balance; so I'm not hurting too badly. But every medical expense, whether legitimate or not, goes to swell the national medical bill and thus the medical insurance bill. Medicare then raises its rates or reduces its benefits, and the private insurers do the same.

Now, my impression that this fellow with the beard was riding the gravy train is only an impression. I don't know, and I have no satisfactory way of finding out. Besides, when I'm a patient I want to have everything possible going for me. So I'm not going to inquire whether bills are padded, and I'm not going to shop around (as the Reagan Administration thinks I should) to get the cheapest rates.

You might think my GP [general practitioner] blameworthy for sending in all those specialists. Yet put yourself in his shoes. Suppose he doesn't call in all the specialists and suppose they don't order all the blood tests and X-rays and CAT scans and MRIs [magnetic-resonance-imaging units]. Then suppose I wind up with a serious ailment that might have been avoided. As I keep telling you, I'm a mild-mannered man and I'd probably not sue, but plenty of others would. So to guard against a malpractice suit,

[2]Reprint of an article contributed by George P. Brockway to *The New Leader*. Reprinted with permission of The New Leader D 28 '87, copyright © The American Conference on International Affairs, Inc.

the GP orders every specialist in sight. Of course, peer review might be able to do something about this problem, and for all I know it does; but I'm sure it's not easy.

Insurance companies keep trying to get legislatures to limit the amount of damages that can be collected, or to outlaw claims for pain and suffering. This seems to me an unreasonable solution. Malpractice does occur, and accidents do occur. Should I lose the use of my right hand because of an incompetent or accidental slip of a surgeon's knife, I'd not be "made whole," as the lawyers say, by a free night in the hospital (less legal fees). If the doctors can't afford high malpractice premiums, and the insurance companies can't afford to lower them, I can't see any course short of turning the whole thing over to the government. As Charles O. Gregory argued in a wise and witty book entitled *Torts and Retorts,* all sorts of personal injury claims (torts) should be the responsibility of the State.

A leading theme in the history of Western law has been the gradual transfer to the State of rights and duties that in more primitive civilizations were private. In ancient Greece, triremes were built not at State expense but at the expense of rich men chosen by lot for the honor. In late medieval Italy, all families of any consequence maintained private militia, like the followers of the Montagues and the Capulets, and competed in building lofty military towers that would enable them to overawe their neighbors. San Gimignano, a town of no great size, had 70 such towers, 14 of which still stand. (A civilizing step was the passage of a municipal law—a zoning ordinance—prohibiting towers beyond a certain height.) For centuries, the detection and punishment of crime was solely the obligation of the injured. Fairly late, the impersonal judgment of God was rendered via trial by battle and trial by ordeal. Secular public enforcement of criminal law is a relatively new idea.

In the same way, health care is gradually shifting its ground. The notion of fee for service is already being compromised by the movement to shame doctors into accepting approved fees. It's not too much to hope that we may eventually have the sense to adopt the better European systems.

A step in this direction has been taken by Massachusetts. Cynics say it is a calculated maneuver in Governor Michael S. Dukakis' play for the [1988] Democratic Presidential nomination. Giving the Duke the benefit of the doubt, I still think his scheme is an example of what Samuel Johnson said about good intentions and the road to hell.

There are close to 6 million residents of Massachusetts and almost 700,000 of them have no health insurance. I must admit I'm astonished that so few are not covered. About two-thirds of the uninsured are employed or are dependents of people who are employed. The Governor proposes to narrow the gap by requiring all employers to insure their employees, with the state picking up the relatively small balance. Clearly what makes the scheme attractive is Massachusetts' present unemployment rate, said to be less than 2 per cent, since the drain on the Commonwealth fisc won't require dramatically higher taxes. Before the days of high-tech, when Massachusetts' unemployment rate was one of the highest in the country, the scheme wouldn't have seemed so painless.

That brings us to the second problem. Whatever the condition of business, universal employer-financed health insurance has a damping effect on employment. Once additional employees cost you several hundred dollars apiece beyond their pay, you're not so cavalier about hiring them. (Social Security taxes, right now, work to discourage employers in this way; they're also heavily regressive on employees.)

Just because we've stumbled along this half century with a far from perfect Social Security system doesn't mean that more of the same won't hurt us. In *The Next Left* Michael Harrington argues persuasively that piling payroll taxes on payroll taxes was largely responsible for the high unemployment that contributed to the failure of Socialist President François Mitterand's program in France. It could happen here.

Aside from Workmen's Compensation, medical insurance has no special connection with employment. In a more civilized nation, all such protection would be a national responsibility, met out of the general revenue without the intervention of insurance companies, private or public. The tax bill might then seem higher, but the drain on the common wealth would be very much less, and the salutary effect on the general welfare would be very much greater.

For this reason I'm not passionately interested in HR 2470, the bill the House has passed limiting some catastrophic medical expenses to $2,000 a year. And speaking personally, although our medical bills will be many times $2,000 this year, HR 2470 will not, as I understand it, benefit us in the slightest. The insurance company that wrote the group policy I've mentioned will get all the benefit, and we will have to pay maybe $1,160 a year in increased Medicare premiums. The insurance companies that will be hit are the TV bandits—if their bemused subscribers have the sense to drop them as utterly useless as well as scandalously expensive.

Those committed to laissez-faire insurance complain that HR 2470 provides for a sliding scale of premiums. Since this tops out at an Adjusted Gross Income of $14,166, my objection is not that it is progressive, but that it is not progressive enough. It is not reasonable for anyone with an annual gross income of $14,166 to be put in the same class with David Rockefeller, or even with me.

The third medical problem is the hundreds of thousands— soon to be tens of millions—of senior citizens who can no longer take care of themselves. In the good old days, before there were such things as senior citizens, the old folks moved in with the young folks, or possibly had a spinster daughter move in with them. In either case, the elders were able to give their adult offspring the benefit of their long-accumulated wisdom, driving the off-spring to spring up the wall. In many a home, something approaching *The Tragedy of King Lear* was re-enacted. Yet both generations took some comfort in the fact that the elders were not a public charge. Where, for lack of family support, they were, the public poor house took over.

All this has changed, for reasons we're all familiar with: Family ties are looser today; individual pride is stronger; the expected life span is very much longer; bottom-line-conscious employers are quick to replace high-priced and slowed-down old hands with eager beginners; and medical research has rendered many diseases incapacitating rather than killing.

These changes lead to the matter of nursing homes and how to pay for them. They are not paid for by Medicare or by most commercial health insurance. They are paid for by Medicaid, but only at the expense of near-pauperization. The rules are complicated, and complicated revisions are daily suggested; yet it remains at best a disheartening and dishonoring process, especially for the middle class that has worked hard for independence. What's to do about it?

Actually a simple solution suggests itself. Instead of forcing pauperization before entry into a nursing home, apply the force at the end. That is, if it is reasonable for the government to exact as full payment as possible for nursing home care, let it do so from the patients' estates after death, not from their reserves. They would thus be able to retain the hope, however slim, of being able one day to take care of themselves again, outside the confines of the nursing home. Moreover, they would be spared the shame of pauperizing both themselves and their spouses, or the alternative heart-wrench of unwanted divorce in order to protect the independence of the noninstitutionalized partner.

Obviously it would be difficult to devise regulations that would forestall the temptation to diddle the government in one way or another. But the same difficulty obtains under the present system. Obviously, too, it would cost the government something to have to wait for its money. On the other hand, the money, when the government finally got it, would tend to be greater, for there would be no need for most of the exceptions that now limit Medicaid's claim on a patient's means.

Finally, some will object that my plan would deprive offspring of their rightful inheritance. To them I reply: (1) The heirs of patients pauperized as a condition of Medicaid inherit little or nothing as it is; and (2) I'm not one to do battle for the right of inheritance, anyhow. In fact, I join economists as various as [Frederich August Von] Hayek and [John Maynard] Keynes in thinking the right might well be abolished. But that is another question.

THE HEALTH CARE COST CRISIS[3]

A woman in El Paso, Texas, slipped and fell on a patch of ice. She broke her ankle—a rather minor accident. Her rather major medical bill came to a whopping $7,000.

In 1984 Americans spent $387 billion on medical care, or $1,580 for each person in the United States—some 11% of the gross national product. Compare that with a total of $190 billion,

[3]Reprint of an article by Gregory Hoelscher, former professor of economics and currently an economist at a major New York bank, and Carolyn Lochhead, a freelance journalist specializing in economics. From *Consumer's Research Magazine*, 69:17–21. O '86. Copyright © 1986 Consumer's Research Magazine. Reprinted by Permission.

or $854 for each person in 1978—only 8.8% of GNP. Medicare
and Medicaid together are the fourth largest item in the federal
budget and consume one-third of all direct federal spending.
According to its own 1984 annual report, Medicare will be broke
by 1991.

In the private sector, evidence of the cost crisis is equally
apparent. Corporate spending on medical care doubled from
1978 to 1984, reaching $77 billion, or one half of total corporate
profits. Joseph Califano, former Health, Education and Welfare
secretary, estimated last fall that medical obligations for the 14
million employees working for the largest private corporations
have reached $2 trillion—exceeding those companies' $1.4 trillion in total assets.

And worse lies ahead. The U.S. population is aging rapidly,
just as medical advances are prolonging life. And health care for
the elderly costs 3.5 times more than for young people.

For under-insured individuals, the price spiral means that a
hospital stay can wipe out a life's savings. For employees and
employers, it means ballooning insurance premiums. For the taxpayer, it means limitless demands on his resources. In short, the
health-care cost spiral is headed toward bankruptcy, and we need
a way out. But how do we get out?

There are two broad strategies for reform of the health-care
system, and they lead in opposite directions. The first extends
government regulation to medical prices. The new Medicare
DRGs, or diagnostic-related groups, use this approach. The other
strategy—the incentive approach—would shift medical choices
and responsibilities to the consumer.

More regulation may seem, at first glance, to be appropriate.
After all, it's the doctors and hospitals who have been raising
prices. But let's go back to 1965, when medical costs began their
upward flight. Not coincidentally, that's also when Medicare and
Medicaid, the two government insurance programs that now cover half of all the nation's medical care, began.

Ten years after Medicare and Medicaid were enacted, hospital
charges had risen 300%. In 1965, Medicare was projected to cost
$9 billion a year by 1990. By 1983, costs had already hit $61 billion.

Why the high costs? Medicare/Medicaid, and Blue Cross/Blue
Shield and private insurance are all so-called third-party programs, which pay most of the medical bill incurred by the
insured. A health-care transaction, such as an operation, then, is

not solely between consumer (patient) and provider (doctor or hospital), but includes a third party. And when a third party pays for health care, it shields both consumer and provider from the price. The extent of this price shield is wide: in 1983, third parties paid for 92% of hospital care and 72% of physicians' services.

Until recently, much third-party insurance was also "first-dollar" coverage, meaning the patient paid little or no deductible or co-payment (a co-payment is the proportion of the total bill paid by the patient, even after the deductible is met). From the first dollar on, the third party paid. So patients and doctors saw little reason to hold down the cost of medical care, because that cost was born by insurers or government.

One of the primary reasons for the spread of private "third-party" coverage is the U.S. tax code. Health-care benefits provided by employers to employees are tax free. So $1,200 in company-provided health benefits buys $1,200 in health care. But if the same $1,200 were paid to an employee in cash, some $300 to $600 would go to federal and state income taxes and Social Security taxes. As a result, the employee could buy just $600 to $900 in health care on his own, not $1,200.

The effect of this tax incentive favoring company-paid insurance is far-reaching. Large businesses now pay a substantial portion of their payroll in the form of health benefits. Chrysler, for instance, attributes 10% of the total cost of producing K-cars to employee health benefits. Yet companies have little incentive to pressure their insurers to cut costs, because any insurance savings paid out as higher wages are taxable income. The tax law also discourages co-payment and deductibles while encouraging paid-in-full benefits.

Moreover, until the early '80s, most third-party programs used a "cost-plus" system of payment. (Many health bills paid through private insurers such as Blue Cross/Blue Shield are still reimbursed on a cost-plus basis.) Under such a system, hospitals and doctors are automatically reimbursed for practically any service they provide. Assured of payment, they oblige. Indeed, revenues are greatest when tests, operations, exams and the like are performed in great quantity. Small wonder then that from 1965 to 1970 hospital admission rates rose 25%, the average length of stay increased 50%, and the surgery rate rose 40%. The cost-plus system encouraged doctors and hospitals to *raise* costs, not to lower them.

No less at fault are malpractice suits and the advance of high-cost medical technology used in practicing "defensive medicine." Better for the doctor to order more tests—which insurance will cover automatically—than to risk being sued for negligence. And facing no restraint on using new technology to protect themselves, doctors rely on the "highest ethical standard"—which means do whatever tests or procedures you think might apply, regardless of cost.

Needless to say, with the cost-plus system of providing health care, doctors and hospitals needn't, as in days past, worry about their patients' financial status. Patients don't worry either; often, they don't even see their bills. In fact, because patients have no reason to scrutinize costs, their demand for "costless" health care is unlimited: the lower the price paid by the consumer, the more health care he will demand.

But ultimately consumers *do* pay the bill. They pay it through higher taxes and higher insurance premiums. Some 22% of Medicare's budget comes from general taxes, the rest from the payroll tax, split 50/50 between employers and employees. Last year [1985] the payroll tax took 2.9% of total earnings—by 1995 it will swallow more than 5%. Health insurance premiums now account for almost 5% of consumers' disposable income, as opposed to less than 3% during the 1960s.

Third-party insurance and cost-plus payment have combined to form a shield around consumers and providers, anesthetizing them to prices. This in turn has caused demand and costs to soar. The result is the health-care cost crisis.

To fight this crisis the federal government is turning to new controls—on hospital capacity, on prices, on utilization, and perhaps soon on physicians' fees. The best-known of these controls are the diagnostic-related groups, or DRGs. DRGs establish fees for 468 categories of illnesses for which Medicare reimburses hospitals. Treatment for a fracture has a set price of, say, $3,000. If a hospital charges more, it has to swallow the difference. If the hospital's costs come in below $3,000, it pockets a profit. The DRG system was instituted for 30% of the nation's acute-care hospitals in 1983 and will be completely phased in for Medicare patients by 1988.

Early estimates show that DRGs have cut the government's Medicare costs . . . for now. Hospitals have slashed personnel, supplier prices and lengths of stay. Yet DRGs will probably only make matters much worse. In the longer run, DRGs will actually boost health-care costs *and* lower the quality of treatment, because they reinforce old and create new perverse incentives.

To begin with, patient well-being could all too easily suffer. Hospitals already are discharging patients faster. There are already reports of hospitals that place patients in the highest-paying DRG category. This "DRG-creep" means ailment A soon becomes ailment B.

Paul Ginsberg, a researcher for the Rand Corporation, found that the number of cases placed in higher-cost DRGs rose 8.4% in 1984, twice as much as Medicare administrators expected. And this was before hospitals had much chance to gear up for the new system. Now, hospitals are adding sophisticated computer programs and diagnostic specialists to make sure patients are placed in the "right" DRG (one that reimburses at or above costs). In this respect, DRGs tend only to shift and conceal costs, not lower them.

Perhaps more ominous, DRGs also thwart the development and use of new technology by directing it toward cutting costs rather than benefitting patients. Before DRGs, even the most marginal technical improvements sold quickly. Hospitals could afford not to be discriminating. Yet regulation removes more than excesses. Frank E. Smaule Jr., president of the Health Industry Manufacturers Association, says that with DRGs "research and development will be directed at lower-cost improvements. Quality improvements that also raise costs will come in second."

To solve such problems, Robert Rubin, the architect of DRGs, calls for a "Prospective Payment Assessment Commission" to "evaluate the potential of new technologies to assure that the new regulations don't pose a barrier to possible medical breakthroughs." Clearly, DRG regulation is creating problems that didn't exist before—problems which in turn require more regulation.

But when bureaucrats attempt to squeeze new technology into the DRG corset, the effect could be counterproductive: for example, an expensive, new, magnetic-resonance-imaging technology similar to an X-ray machine has been approved for DRG reimbursement. The new technique is more remunerative than X-rays and CAT scans, so hospitals could easily favor it even for cases where the old techniques would work just as well.

Says Roger Noll, a Stanford University economist who has analyzed the effect of regulation on health care: "This is the classic problem with regulation. When you regulate technology, all kinds of economic perversities get introduced. Some things (such as expensive, but life-saving technology) will be retarded; some things will be unacceptably encouraged (such as high-cost X-rays). Arbitrary accounting principles will drive the pattern of technological change."

Already DRGs are threatening to become a classic regulatory hydra. One regulation begets yet more—cut off one head, and five others sprout. After just two years' experience with DRGs, the General Accounting Office is already in search of ways to stem the problems DRGs have created.

One physician suggested using a "severity index" to curb DRG abuse and protect patients. Government regulators would use the index to determine how patients with varying degrees of illness fit into each of the 468 DRGs while "taking into account the special needs" of each Medicare patient.

This is the crux of the regulatory dilemma: Regulations must be simple in order to be comprehensive, so by their very nature they cannot account for individual needs or foresee technical change, especially in so dynamic a field as medicine. As the regulations mount, they become ever more complex, costly and stifling. The Hospital Association of New York found that, even before DRGs, 25% of a hospital's costs were due solely to government regulation. And yet the government is proposing 6000 more DRG categories for physicians and other professionals.

Further regulation of health care will continue to treat only the symptoms of the crisis, the most dramatic of which is rising costs. At the same time, it will further aggravate the initial ailment.

The health care problem must be attacked at its roots—in the marketplace. By lifting the price shield, created in large part by third-party payments and tax subsidies, consumers must be exposed to actual health care costs. This can be done by taking the *incentives approach,* which is already being used to reduce health care spending in some parts of the country. Its primary goal is to reduce the growth in demand for health care. The incentives approach offers consumers a chance to get low-cost, high-quality care. It also gives providers an incentive to supply the same.

One reform target is tax deductions for employers who provide employee health insurance. With a limit on these, employers and employees would face a higher incentive to monitor insurance costs. Third-party insurers, under pressure from their customers, would in turn have to monitor their costs more closely. Use patterns would quickly change, and providers would be forced to cut costs in order to retain customers. As competition intensified, insurers would begin to extract more favorable terms from providers.

"First-dollar" insurance, already being phased out by many private and public insurers, would become far more expensive and even less popular. Households and employers, taking the full cost of insurance into account, would shoulder more of the cost of routine health care, greatly reducing demand and the pressure on costs. As consumer responsiveness was restored, it would in turn force doctors to begin taking cost into consideration.

Increasing deductibles would, without doubt, severely curb insurance overuse—not only in private insurance, but in Medicare and Medicaid too.

According to a Rand study, people fully covered by health insurance spend 60% more on medical care than those who face even a 5% deductible. Many employers, hit with huge hikes in insurance premiums, have already begun to experiment with selective plans that have larger deductibles or co-payments. One survey shows that private comprehensive medical plans with deductibles of more than $100 increased from 65% to 90% from 1980 to 1984. Even the federal government is getting into the act: Medicare broadened its deductible/co-payment strategy in 1985.

Employers are also exploring alternatives such as health maintenance organizations (HMOs). HMOs are an alternative to fee-for-service coverage—they charge a flat annual fee for all medical services and therefore face a built-in incentive to hold down costs. But HMOs are hardly the only option; because the market has been so tightly regulated, a wide spectrum of alternative delivery systems remains unexplored. These options will give the consumer more freedom to choose an insurance plan that suits his own needs.

One suggestion—proposed in 1980 by Congressmen [Richard] Gephardt and [David] Stockman, and more recently by other legislators—would provide for a multiple choice of insurance plans. Instead of providing tax-free health benefits, employers and Medicare/Medicaid would offer a fixed-dollar subsidy or "voucher" to consumers, which would be at least enough to pay for basic insurance. Consumers would then shop around for the plan that best suits their own medical and financial needs. If the plan they choose is more expensive than the employer or government contribution, they would pay the difference. If less, they would pocket the difference.

Vouchers create a powerful incentive for consumers and through them, providers, to reduce costs. When health expenses are paid out-of-pocket from voucher money, savings—and costs—are more apparent. Consumers will look for the company offering the best deal, and those will be the most cost-efficient companies. This voucher system returns choice to the consumer; he can tailor his health care to his own needs—both physical and financial.

Another key to the incentives approach is to avoid laws that would further distort the insurance market, such as mandated benefits. Required levels of coverage have often been proposed in Congress. Yet an insurer's most effective cost-containment tool is his ability to adjust coverage. Other insurance has built-in mechanisms to curb abuse. Automobile insurers use claim adjusters, require multiple estimates, set fixed cash benefits and set up contracts with providers, such as auto body shops. Health insurers should be allowed to do the same.

One must also examine the supply of health care. If it cannot expand to meet demand, prices will inevitably rise, DRGs or no DRGs. Many supply constraints, such as those that limit the supply of doctors and the use of advertising, can easily be removed, and some have been.

The federal government also erects barriers to competition. It not only subsidizes but "qualifies" HMOs for Medicare patients, so the first qualified HMO in a community gets a sharp competitive edge. Because of federal assistance, HMOs may be crowding out other alternatives.

The government could start cutting its own Medicare costs (much more simply and effectively than DRGs attempt to do) by instituting competitive bidding among providers. In the private sector, contracting is growing rapidly where insurance laws are no barrier.

Health care is swallowing an ever-larger portion of our national income. Part of the rising cost reflects broader coverage and new medical technologies. But the bulk is due to overconsumption of health care and inefficient use of medical resources, caused largely by government regulation and tax policy. More regulation will not cure the old problems, but it will create new ones.

In contrast, the incentives approach will yield lower costs for society and wider choice for consumers. It will allow the government to decide the *level* of support to provide the indigent and the elderly. It does not ask government to set its price or determine how health care is delivered to patients—that decision is best made by doctors, hospitals, and their patients.

The case of a Medicare patient in Texas illustrates the folly of bureaucratic price setting. The federal government's DRG payment for a woman with colon-cancer complications allowed her 5.9 days of hospitalization and less than $2,000 in medical care. But this elderly patient required more than six weeks of care—for which the DRG category does not allow the hospital to be reimbursed. The inflexible rule forces the hospital to skimp on her care (early discharge), cheat on the rules (DRG creep), or cover her excess costs by over-charging other patients. Unfortunately, this is not an isolated case. It is a common result of the regulatory approach to cutting health-care costs.

Rather than imposing complex and ultimately counterproductive schemes to regulate doctors and hospitals, perhaps now it's time to unshackle the consumer. This approach has never really been tried. But the consumer's exercise of free choice can attain what an army of bureaucrats can never hope to: cost-effective medical care for everyone.

MEETING SKYROCKETING HEALTH CARE COSTS[4]

How many times have we heard the statement, "An ounce of prevention is worth a pound of cure"? Shortly after employers felt the sharp pinch of spiraling health care costs in the early 1980's, there emerged various programs designed to prevent accident and illness, both on and off the job. In theory, by altering the lifestyles of employees and their families, many illnesses and accidents could be avoided, thus saving employers a significant portion of their medical insurance expenses.

In most cases, these programs, while well-intentioned, showed

[4]Reprint of an article by Donald Lightfoot, senior vice president, Sedgwick Jones Financial Services in Los Angeles. Reprinted from USA TODAY MAGAZINE, May copyright © 1990 by the Society for the Advancement of Education.

little hard data to support their cost-reduction claims and never really obtained any significant degree of universal acceptance. Without established cost/benefit studies to prove the value of prevention programs, chief financial officers (CFO's) and risk managers turned their attention to other methods of managing their expenses, primarily claims administration enhancements through improved systems, negotiating lower rates with providers, and utilization review programs.

As we enter the 1990's, health care costs are out of control again. Red ink is everywhere for all those involved in this eventual trillion-dollar industry revolution. Moreover, little relief is in sight because the increases—due primarily to rising hospital operating costs for outpatient procedures—are unavoidable.

Hospitals are shifting costs to make up for some of the increased expense of doing business and raising charges dramatically for certain services. As a result, the average charge per hospital stay in 1988 rose 19% from the previous year, even though the average length of stay rose only two percent, according to an EQUICOR survey of 1,863 hospitals nationwide.

With profits continuing to slip for hospitals to near zero, the cost of hospital charges will continue to escalate. There really is only one solution—we must keep people out of hospitals and doctors' offices. This can be done best through employee education and prevention programs that work and have proven to be effective.

Employers of all sizes are coming to realize that virtually all employee benefits—even compensation and productivity—are affected greatly by workers' well-being. Obviously, those who are sick or injured cost employers more than healthy employees do in direct outlays and lost productivity and profitability.

Many of the prevention programs that will be used over the next decade or so haven't even been designed yet. However, the issues they must address already have been determined.

A survey by a national consulting firm found that most CFO's and CEO's who were interviewed placed three topics as top priority in the years ahead: being competitive and productive globally, AIDS, and substance abuse in the workplace.

Most corporations do not have policies to address issues concerning AIDS, despite fear that victims will cause substantial health, accident, and death claims. More than two-thirds of 628 companies surveyed at random by *Fortune* magazine said they were concerned about AIDS, yet had developed no specific corporate policy on the disease.

According to former Surgeon General C. Everett Koop, the AIDS programs that have been developed, although few in number, are good. More are needed, however. He suggested a corporate prevention plan which not only provides information and education on the AIDS virus, but, in addition, involves corporate policy guidelines on how to treat the disease in the workplace and the legal ramifications for all parties concerned, with periodic updates to keep current.

Similar preventive packages should, and are, being developed for drug and alcohol abuse in the workplace. Employers need better outreach programs to their employees to help control this illness, which continues to invade the lives of so many and drives down corporate profits.

There is another preventive measure which deserves special attention, one that addresses the areas of major concern for corporate America: health care and workers compensation costs, and global competitiveness and profitability. It is a simple flexibility stretching regimen for business and home, which as proven to be successful in reducing injuries, lost work, and compensation expenses. As a result, productivity increases and employee morale is enhanced.

Designed and marketed in 1982, the Athletes in Industry prevention program aims at the source of 50% of workers compensation and 25% of health claims—sprains and strains of the torso, with specific emphasis on the lower back. Results have been impressive in reducing workers compensation cases, and we expect the same to be true for health claims when they are tracked. To my knowledge, there is no other prevention process available that can impact both workers compensation and health care so effectively.

At Blue Cross of California, 25% of their clients' off-the-job group health claims are related to sprains and strains of the torso. For the most part, these are preventable and can be controlled with some simple employee education and stretching instruction.

It stands to reason that employee benefit costs can be impacted favorably for those employers participating in the Athletes in Industry prevention program, since it stresses on- and off-the-job flexibility stretching. With heavy rate increases predicted from workers compensation and health care carriers, employers are finding that this plan addresses both financial concerns.

When employers make the commitment to this prevention program, Athletes in Industry consultants go to work with the firms' personnel to introduce the idea to supervisors and employees; explain to them how flexibility stretching works to prevent injuries both on and off the job; train team leaders; implement the flexibility stretching exercises; follow up throughout the year with performance measurement and support; and provide a monthly newsletter to each participant that reinforces healthy lifestyles and safety. All workers then do the static stretching exercises, with management support, for six to eight minutes at the beginning of each workday.

The success of this preventive measure is in its simplicity, packaging, and tracked effectiveness. Every level of employee can and does participate in the stretching. Typically, employers initiate the routine to a number of their employees, with expansion to other members of the workforce. The cost depends on the number of participants, but the first-year price generally would be around two percent of the monthly health care premium, or $18–20 per year per employee. Saving one back injury—which, on average, costs more than $10,000—would pay for this prevention program for 300 participants for two years.

With significant percentages of workers compensation and group health claims occurring due to sprains and strains of the torso, it has been proven that the cost/benefit ratio associated with this stretching program will be at least four-to-one or better. The results will vary, depending upon the corporation's industry and past injury and medical claim history.

Corporations that have implemented this stretching routine report they would do it all over again without considering any financial gains because of improved worker awareness and attitude. Further, they indicate that, unlike other fitness and exercise classes where relatively few participate, virtually all employees offered the stretch program do the routine daily, and they "have fun" doing it.

The trend toward more proven prevention programs that address the major issues of today will become a way of corporate life. The economic impact of back injuries, for example, is too great to ignore.

A nationwide survey of CEO's found that 67% plan to institute or expand the health prevention idea during the next two years. The double-barreled rate hike from workers compensation and health care insurance has forced many corporate decision-makers to institute prevention programs that work both on and off the job. No longer is there justification for "fluff" wellness programs that accomplish little for too few of their employees.

Health care in America has evolved from the traditional fee-for-service delivery system, which essentially gave providers a blank check, to a cost-containment approach, to managed health care concepts. Nevertheless, expenses continue to soar, and providers find new methods of "beating the system."

Thus, the next logical step has to be prevention. Our mission must be to keep people healthy and out of the health care delivery system. Only then will skyrocketing monetary outlays finally be controlled.

II. HEALTH CARE PROVIDERS

EDITOR'S INTRODUCTION

What used to be called the "medical profession" a generation ago is now sometimes referred to as "the medical-industrial complex." It is a huge industry, larger even than the defense industry, that has brought not only greater efficiency and profit but also greater impersonalization and stress to those who dispense medical service to the public. The traditional family doctor who made house calls has been replaced by the staff physician in a large hospital, perhaps a chain hospital, where the profit margin has been carefully calculated. Section Two of this volume addresses the changed world of American medicine. In the opening article, reprinted from *Time*, staffwriter Nancy R. Gibbs discusses the new doctor-patient relationship, one too-often marked by distrust or uncertainty on each side. The doctor is harrassed by the threat of malpractice suits, the pressure of public expectations, and the endless paperwork required by insurers, government regulators, lawyers, consultants, and risk managers. Small wonder, despite the high incomes commanded by physicians, that applications to medical schools have declined sharply in the late 1980s.

The next piece, by Dena Seidin in *Commonweal*, examines the malpractice insurance crisis in the medical profession, the cost of which is passed on to patients through higher doctors' bills. Malpractice insurance, which may cost $50,000 or more a year, has been a special hardship for young doctors just starting out. In a number of cases, they have moved their practice to states like Indiana, where law suits are infrequent and thus malpractice premiums are relatively low, largely because stringent state laws control the nature and amounts of awards. But the migration of doctors to such areas may result in a shortage of physicians in other areas. In another development, physicians are forsaking private practice for salaried posts with institutions—profit-making hospital chains, HMOs, medical schools, and teaching hospitals. The article also examines the trend toward "defensive medicine," excessive diagnostic procedures and testing that added $42 billion to the national medical bill in 1986 alone. Finally, Seiden discusses moves toward reform in malpractice litigation, particularly the move to put a cap on "pain and suffering" awards in the courts.

Next, in an article from *Newsweek,* James N. Baker notes the drop in applications to medical schools—by 26% since 1975, with an additional 10% for the entering class of 1987. As applications from white males decline, women and minority groups would seem likely to have larger representations in the medical schools in the future. A related article in *Time* by Christine Gorman surveys the situation of the nursing profession. Nursing schools have also reported dramatic declines in enrollment at a time when the need for nurses is greater than ever. Overworked and underpaid, nurses will need stronger incentives, particularly larger salaries and a more clearly defined professional status, if nursing is to continue to be a strong component of national health care.

The next two articles, both from *Society,* deal with hospitals. In the first, Geraldine Dallek examines the inception and subsequent dramatic growth of for-profit hospitals, including Humana and the Hospital Corporation of America (HCA). For-profit hospitals charge higher rates than public hospitals and earn enormous profits, adding to the staggering $400 billion spent annually in the country on health care. They have been characterized generally as businesslike concern for the profit margin, but less interest in providing care for the economically disadvantaged. By serving only patients able to pay their rates, for-profit hospitals have created a situation where the indigent or uninsured are "dumped" onto non-profit or public hospitals, creating a two-tiered system of medical treatment. The marketplace mentality of the for-profit hospitals, Dallek concludes, allows "corporate medicine to distort our medical care system into one that costs us a great deal even while it serves a diminishing share of people." In the second article from *Society,* Robert G. Hughes and Philip R. Lee look at the condition of the public hospitals. Worst off are the urban public hospitals, often with antiquated physical plants, which must accept a growing caseload of uninsured patients while depending on the largesse of local and state governments that are themselves hard pressed economically. The great question for the public hospitals, as Hughes and Lee point out, is how they are to manage their survival and still fulfill their mandate to serve the poor and the disadvantaged.

SICK AND TIRED[1]

"I do not know a single thoughtful and well-informed person," George Bernard Shaw once said, "who does not feel that the tragedy of illness at present is that it delivers you helplessly into the hands of a profession which you deeply mistrust."

That sentiment is mild compared with some of today's reviews. Doctor bashing has become a blood sport. To judge by the popular press, which generally lacks Shaw's subtlety, too many physicians who are not magicians are charlatans. The air of the operating room, where once the doctor was sovereign, is now so dense with the second guesses of insurers, regulators, lawyers, consultants and risk managers that the physician has little room to breathe, much less heal. Small wonder that the doctor-patient relationship, once something of a sacred covenant, has been infected by the climate in which it grows.

All this means that it is simply harder to be a doctor now than it was a generation ago: harder to master the art and the craft, harder to practice, harder to savor the natural pleasures of healing. Patients loudly long for the days of chummy family doctors and personalized care, when Marcus Welby would make everyone well. But it turns out that the distress is mutual, the frustration shared. Many patients may be surprised to learn that the doctors are suffering too. Listen to them tell it:

• "Once most people treated me as a friend and a confidant," recalls Boyd McCracken Sr., 65, a family practitioner from Greenville, Ill. (pop. 5,000), who remembers making late-night house calls. "These days the malpractice threat has created a definite wedge between a physician and some of his patients."

• "I think patients have become consumers," says Robert Rogers, an ophthalmologist in Pompano Beach, Fla. "They are no longer interested in their doctor, who has perhaps been their doctor for five, six, ten years. They are really interested in what it's going to cost them. It's just like they're going shopping at the local supermarket."

• "I get no sense they trust me," says Jonathan Licht, a San Diego neurologist. "You tell them, 'You're O.K.' They say, 'No,

[1]Reprint of an article by *Time* staff writer, Nancy R. Gibbs. Reprinted by permission from *Time*, 134: 48-53. Jl 31'89. Copyright © 1989 Time Inc.

I'm not O.K. I think I have a brain tumor.' Then they keep asking, 'How do you really know?'"

All across the U.S., among family doctors and brain surgeons, in large cities and small towns, the tensions are growing. Perhaps many doctors just miss their pedestals and the days when their patients were more respectful and their diagnoses unchallenged. But the soreness may also reflect the stresses and strains of a profession in transition. Nothing in medicine is stationary: the blinding speed of technological advances, the splintering effects of specialization, the onset of medical consumerism, the threat of malpractice suits have all bruised the doctor-patient relationship in recent years.

There are rich ironies here. Never have doctors been able to do so much for their patients, and rarely have patients seemed so ungrateful. Eighty years ago, a sick man who consulted his physician had roughly a fifty-fifty chance of benefiting from the encounter. The doctor's cheery manner and solicitous style were compensation for the uncertainty of a cure. "Medicine originally was mainly talk," says Sidney Wolfe, a physician who directs the Public Citizen Health Research Group in Washington, "and very little effective diagnosis and treatment."

Compare that with the prospects of today's patient: what was once miraculous is now mundane. The flutist has her severed hand sewn back on. The man with the transplanted heart goes skiing. As a society, Americans are living longer and well and with less to fear from diseases that ravaged whole generations. Life expectancy has jumped during this century from 47 to 75 years. And yet the physicians, victims of their own success, are finding that however swift the advance of medical knowledge, it is still outpaced by public expectations. "The public thinks that all diseases should be treatable, all disabilities reparable," observes John Stoeckle, chief of the medical clinics at Massachusetts General Hospital. "And there should be no pain and suffering."

So naturally, the public is far from content. In part the problem lies with the failure of the profession and the government to police medicine adequately, since the stakes could not be higher. If a stockbroker is incompetent, his client may lose his savings; if a doctor is negligent, his patient may lose his vision, his memory, his mobility or his life. Though the public, the government and the physicians themselves have become more vigilant, the persistent stories of medical mishaps continue to take their toll on patient confidence.

The anger and suspicion toward doctors are easy to measure, even without reading the tabloids or watching *Geraldo* for the latest tally of medical misdeeds. When the American Medical Association conducts surveys of public attitudes toward physicians, it finds a troubling loss of faith. Even people who esteem their own physicians often deride the profession as a whole. In 1987, 37% of those polled did not believe doctors take a genuine interest in their patients. Only 45% believed doctors "usually explain things well to their patients."

A doctor's words may speak louder than actions, but every patient hears them differently, and doctors end up feeling they cannot win. When Cincinnati receptionist Doris Roetting had a mastectomy in the fall of 1987, her surgeon assured her that she was recuperating nicely. Her oncologist, however, was a bit more explicit, to Roetting's dismay. He quietly explained that she had a 90% chance of being alive in five years and an 80% chance of surviving ten years. Some patients might have been grateful for such candor; Roetting went home in tears. "I think everybody who has cancer knows there is a chance they can have it again," she says. "These doctors should show a little more finesse."

Tact and tenderness may be a lot to expect from someone who must spend roughly twelve years learning the trade, work impossible hours, be available to patients day and night, keep abreast of changing technology and live a peaceable life while constantly dealing with death. "The patient wants the best of both worlds," charges Lester King, a Chicago physician and medical historian. "He wants the knowledge and precision of the most advanced science, and the care and concern of the old-fashioned practitioner."

For more and more doctors, that is just too much to ask. They feel the wrath of their patients and realize the job is not going to get any easier. A March 1986 survey of physicians in the Minneapolis-St. Paul area found that nearly two-thirds of them were "pessimistic about their professional futures," and a like number said they would not want their children to go into medicine. Applications to medical schools for the 1988–89 school year declined 15% from 1986–87, reflecting a contagious concern about the profession's future.

As ambivalence and hostility divide doctors and patients, medical experts are struggling to explain the troubled relationship and find ways to revive it. Some of the conflict arises from human nature. How can doctors feel comfortable when patients come into the office prepared to sue them for everything they own? How can patients trust a doctor who has a clear financial interest in prescribing expensive, intrusive and perhaps unnecessary therapies? When doctors disagree, how can a patient know whom to believe? Both sides recognize that the demands of treatment have changed in ways guaranteed to alienate doctor and patient.

The most obvious source of friction is the new technologies that enter into every stage of treatment. Since the end of World War II, as the science of medicine rapidly evolved, the craft overtook the art. Many physicians regret that they now spend far more time testing than talking, which may make for more accurate treatment but less personal care. The race to stay abreast of each new development can consume a doctor's every waking moment. "Technologies have put a kind of emotional moat between doctor and patient," laments David Rogers, professor of medicine at Cornell University Medical College. Some tests, particularly the CAT scan and colonoscopy, not only frighten but dehumanize patients by reducing the body to an intricate piece of machinery.

Doctors often find they can do more but explain less, leaving their patients with the impression that treatment is not to be understood, rather to be suffered. The doctor, for his part, may want to reassure the patient, but balks at taking the time to deliver a discourse on molecular biology. "You have to be tolerant," says Lake Forest, Ill., cardiologist Jay Alexander. "You have to be able to answer questions, and it's got to be an answer that the patient is able to understand. Twenty years ago, I imagine, less explanation would have been necessary." The suspense and confusion weigh heavily on patients and their families. Author Norman Cousins and his followers believe lack of concern for the patient's state of mind can actually cause physical harm. "At its worst," argues Cousins, "it's a form of malpractice."

Yet keeping patients informed becomes ever harder when each test is performed by a different technician in a different building, with no one wanting ultimate responsibility. For Josefina Ponce, a day-care worker in Los Angeles, it took four visits and twelve doctors to have one gallbladder operation. "I saw one doctor in the emergency room, then a second doctor," she recalls. "On my second visit, I saw three different doctors who knew nothing about my case. I was told what my surgery date would be, and I said I wanted to meet my doctor. But I was told there would be five doctors, and it could be any one of them."

Those who, like Ponce, lament the anonymous quality of their treatment reflect a second revolution in patient care, the rise of the medical-industrial complex. Every bit as important as the advances in technology are the means of delivering them and deciding who should pay. Instead of an individual doctor seeing his regular patients in the privacy of his office, the typical encounter now occurs in the thick of a vast corporate hierarchy that monitors every decision and may weigh in against it. Marketing medicine has become very big business.

As costs have risen, the past decade has seen an explosion in prepaid, "managed" care. More than half of all physicians work in some kind of group practice, most commonly a health-maintenance organization. Patients pay a flat annual fee in exchange for care that is provided by HMO member doctors. As private corporations, many HMOs can be quite profitable—so long as their patients do not get too sick. The number of patients enrolled in HMOs has doubled in the past five years, to 32 million, often at the urging of cost-conscious employers. The goals: efficiency through greater competition, lower costs, accountability and better preventive care.

But the results may be mixed. Patients relinquish much of their freedom to choose who will treat them, and can be lost in a shuffle between rotating doctors. The physicians, meanwhile, are transformed from professionals into employees, with a duty to serve not only the interests of their patients but the demands of the corporation as well. "They're asking physicians to pay for their decisions," says internist Madeleine Neems in Lake Bluff, Ill. "That's a terrible concept. When you analyze whether or not a patient needs an expensive test, a lot of times it's not a clear-cut yes or no. I don't want my finances tied into those decisions."

Doctors resent spending extra time with patients who demand exhaustive explanations or who merely exercise their hypochondria. "If you have to spend twice as much time because a patient's assertive and he wants to ask questions, it's certainly difficult to bill for that period of time," says cardiologist Alexander. "Lawyers and accountants don't have third parties or government agencies looking over their shoulders to determine whether their billings are fair." Patients understandably take a spare-no-expense attitude toward their health, but that is not a philosophy likely to keep a medical company in the black.

Physicians and patients who are not part of an HMO have found their lives affected too. The government (as the largest health insurer) and the private insurance companies have tried to cap medical costs by deciding in advance how much a particular treatment should cost and balking at anything above that amount. Many doctors can no longer decide how often they see a patient, when one can be hospitalized, or even what drugs may be prescribed. Those decisions are now in the hands of third parties, hands that have never touched the patient directly.

Medicare and insurance-company guidelines, for example, forbid cardiologists to hospitalize patients for a coronary angiogram unless the patient is desperately ill. Otherwise, it must be done on an outpatient basis. As a result, Los Angeles cardiology consultant Stephen Berens sometimes has his frail or elderly patients take a room in a nearby hotel the night before the procedure. If he decides the patient needs a temporary pacemaker during the angiogram, he often implants the device but does not charge for it, because the Medicare system denies payment except in cases of very obvious need. "To make them approve it, I'd have to exaggerate the risk of going without it," he says. Berens would once have charged $200 for the pacemaker; now he absorbs the cost.

More than a doctor's pride and cash flow may be at stake. Some physicians warn that the need to make rapid decisions, see more patients and control costs could result in faulty diagnoses. Promising but expensive treatments cannot be provided to everyone who needs them, so what is to prevent reserving such care for the rich? The new pressures on hospital care have also affected the way young doctors are trained. Doctors lose the sense of satisfaction that comes from having a personal relationship with patients and helping them through crises, since hospital stays are shorter, patients are sicker, and treatment time is more rushed.

Not only have the scientific and organizational landscapes of medicine changed; so too has the social and economic climate in which physicians practice. In order to sustain public support and federal funds, the medical community trumpets triumphs with abandon. Hospitals spent more than $1.3 billion last year on marketing and advertising. Small wonder that even the desperately sick are surprised when they are not cured. "The whole idea is false," argues author Richard Selzer, a retired surgeon in New Haven, Conn. "No one has ever got off the planet alive. The natural course is to be born, to flourish, to dwindle and to die. Yet the medical profession has encouraged people to think of the natural course as an adversary, to be fought off until the bitter end. Of course, doctors cannot live up to the expectations they have aroused."

Physicians certainly cannot hope to satisfy patients who, instructed by the consumer movement, have come to view medicine as a commodity like any other, despite the fact that it is unlike any other. Once people would no more price-shop for a doctor than they would for a church. But today some patients switch doctors for as little as a $5 saving on the price of a visit.

"You can be a mediocre doctor and discount your fees enough to have all the business you want," observes James T. Galyon, an orthopedic surgeon in Memphis, "rather than trying to be a very fine doctor and achieving a professional reputation that will cause other doctors to refer patients to you. The loser in the long run is the patient."

Other patients are shopping not for savings but for status. This inspires physicians to spend valuable time on self-promotion and merchandising, not skills that contribute materially to patient care. "My feeling was that if you're a decent physician giving decent service, that's really all you should have to do," says Florida ophthalmologist Robert Rogers, who has hired a business consultant to help manage his practice. "But patients don't seem to want that. They like the flashy stuff. They like to see your name in print. They like to see you lecturing."

In an effort to be educated consumers, today's patients read books with titles like *What Your Doctor Didn't Learn in Medical School* and *Take This Book to the Hospital with You*. The message is that a smart patient is an informed patient, who challenges a doctor's authority rather than submits uncritically to the physician's will and whims. Yet that approach rubs raw against a basic instinct. Patients want to trust their doctors, to view them as benign and authoritative. Even those who privately question a doctor's decisions may be loath to express dissent. Doctors admit that an aggressive or challenging patient can be very irritating. "When you can, under certain circumstances, play God, you sometimes tend to behave like you are God," says Cornell's David Rogers. "The enormous satisfaction of being able to help a lot of people makes you impatient with those who question your judgment."

The ultimate price of inflated expectations and consumerist attitudes is the treacherous legal reality that confronts doctors today. Anything short of perfection becomes grounds for penalty. And once again, while it is the doctor who must pay the high insurance premiums and fend off the suits in court, the patient eventually pays a price. The annual number of malpractice suits filed has doubled in the past decade and ushered in the era of defensive medicine and risk managers. No single factor has done more to distance physicians from patients than the possibility that a patient may one day put a doctor on the witness stand.

Manhattan cardiologist Arthur Weisenseel remembers the elderly woman who arrived in Mount Sinai Hospital's emergency room having suffered a heart attack and battling pneumonia. A man and a woman hovered by her bedside, and the emergency staff assumed they were worried relatives. Then the man pulled out a yellow pad, asked for the correct spelling of Weisenseel's last name and identified himself as the family lawyer. "I kind of lost it that day, and I told him to get out," Weisenseel recalls. "That may have been the most distressing situation I've had in 22 years of practice."

The impact of possible litigation is felt long before a patient sets foot in the doctor's office. Some physicians, like Linda Bolton, a pediatrician in Birmingham, Mich., try to screen out potential problems. "It really dictates what happens at the office. If I feel I have people who are litigious, I prefer not to take them as patients." In the past, she has fixed her rates only after she has been notified how much she will have to pay for malpractice insurance.

The costs of practice have driven out hordes of doctors altogether. According to a 1987 survey by the American College of Obstetrics and Gynecology, 1 out of 8 U.S. obstetricians has left the field because of the malpractice threat. Those who manage to stay in business may feel forced to practice a kind of medicine that assumes every patient is a prospective litigant. Such defensive tactics are antithetical to compassionate care: the doctor ends up being afraid of someone he or she wants to help, cautious about trying attractive new treatments and emotionally aloof from someone in need of emotional support.

Doctors recognize a vicious circle here, but there are indications of a possible break. In 1988 for the first time in more than a decade, medical malpractice suits abated. Claims settlements were down $100 million from the 1987 high of $4.2 billion. In response, several major insurers have reduced their premiums. On the basis of studies showing that physicians who know their patients well over a long period are less likely to be sued, more doctors are looking for ways to avoid the fearful, adversarial climate that prompts them to retreat emotionally—which ends up making a suit more likely. "Many malpractice suits come because people are angry at their doctors for not communicating," says Cornell's Rogers. Consumer advocate Michael Rooney of the People's Medical Society agrees: "It's when they feel they've been hurt or betrayed that they sue."

The relationship is actually poisoned on both sides. Patients may insist on the most conscientious care and yet balk at the battery of tests that doctors order to cover themselves. "You come in for an ingrown toenail, and they turn you inside out giving you all kinds of tests that you don't need," says columnist Ann Landers, who receives complaints from all concerned. "The bill is horrendous. The doctors want to be able to prove that they didn't miss anything. It makes people mad, and I don't blame them."

Even as natural a procedure as giving birth has been greatly distorted by the epidemic of lawsuits. "Mothers believe that all babies should be born perfect," observes Massachusetts General's Stoeckle, and here the bond of doctor and patient may be most fragile. Doctors order expensive tests and uncomfortable procedures as protection against future suits. The costs to expectant parents are exorbitant, and discomfort during delivery is heightened: nearly one-quarter of all U.S. births are currently by caesarean section, which can be less risky to the baby than vaginal delivery and makes the doctor less vulnerable in court.

Finally, there are those who argue that litigation actually slows the progress of medicine. "Innovative techniques don't get used very often for this reason," says George Miller, an orthopedic surgeon in Washington, N.C., who last year won a malpractice suit that had dragged on for "eight long years." Doctors find themselves taking a more rote approach, what some call "cookbook medicine." By following standard procedures as much as possible, the physician may hope to avoid any controversy that might arise in court—and thus steers clear of promising, if less proven technologies and treatments.

The combination of these factors—the welter of technology, the intrusions of corporate medicine, the high expectations of patients and the threat of malpractice—has cast a pall on the practice of many older physicians. "I detect a certain despondency among doctors my age, in their later 50s," says Memphis surgeon Galyon. "They will frequently say something to the effect, 'I'm glad I'm this far in my profession and not starting out.'"

Oddly enough, many young physicians do not feel the same way and still see in medicine a career of compassion and challenge, despite its loss of luster in recent years. Their attitudes may reflect new priorities in many medical schools. Traditionally, med school, internship and residency were a notorious, competitive ordeal that all but guaranteed less humane doctors. "It makes book learning and grade getting their yardstick, not kindness, gentleness and taking care of people," says Dr. E. Grey Dimond, founder of the School of Medicine at the University of Missouri at Kansas City and a leader in humanistic medicine.

That may be changing, thanks to some innovative programs that are challenging the conventional curriculum. The most visible experiment, following an example pioneered at Missouri, was launched at Harvard Medical School in 1985. The goal of Harvard's New Pathway Program was to focus from the very first day on the doctor-patient relationship, rather than rely solely on textbook learning. "Even in an era that is overlaid by science and technology," says Harvard Professor Ronald Arky, "doctoring still involves an intimate, close contact with the patient, and somehow that was being pushed out." Small groups of students work closely with a physician and meet with patients on hospital wards almost immediately, in an effort to mix basic science with clinical decision making. Course work draws not only on science but also on literature, history, anthropology and sociology.

As more hospitals and universities increase the emphasis on the doctor-patient relationship, there are signs that attitudes are changing. When humanistic courses were introduced in the 1970s, high-powered students resisted what they viewed as soft science. "Now the students see that the shine on their shingle is affected by what people think of them as human beings," says author Cousins. The profession is attracting a different kind of student: many are less concerned with accumulating wealth for its own sake and more comfortable with patients who ask questions and challenge authority. "It's a much more difficult field now," says Dr. Matthew Conolly at UCLA. "I think we'll see a different set of motivations."

Doctors and patients alike may look forward to the day when better relations mean better care. A strong bond makes it easier for doctors to craft their therapy to the patient's needs. More cynically, some experts predict that competition among doctors will force a more humane approach as a selling point. Finally, the problem of reimbursement could be relieved if insurers came to value a good doctor-patient relationship and were willing to allow doctors more discretion. Says consumer advocate Rooney: "It's a recognition that, in the long run, it may be more important to talk to someone at age 28 than it is to clean out their arteries at 78."

In the end, however, the struggle between caring and curing is not likely to be resolved by invention or innovation. The next generation of doctors may appreciate that medicine is a fine art of human care; their patients may accept the constraints on physicians and resist the temptation to blame them for an absence of miracles. But even if relations ease, the challenges to patients and doctors will still grow. The practice of medicine, though it may become ever more precise, will never again be simple, never cheap and never magic.

THE MALPRACTICE MUDDLE[2]

The medical profession is once again in a "malpractice crisis." The last occurred a decade ago with an attendant fanfare of protests, demonstrations, strikes, and some legislation. The current crisis differs from that of 1975. At that time, the established insurance companies which provided malpractice insurance to physicians simply withdrew from the field, refusing to underwrite liability insurance at any premium price. The crisis now focuses on the extraordinary rise in the cost of premiums being considered by state insurance departments for largely physician-owned medical liability insurance companies (the professionally preferred term for malpractice). These were the companies established in the wake of the 1975 tumult, to provide coverage and to protect physicians against the existing firms' administrative costs, profit margins, etc. Many of these companies are now being found by the various state insurance departments to have inadequate reserves to meet the increasing severity and frequency of suits and awards. Hence, the proposed premium rises, which in New York State would average around 55 percent per carrier according to the most recent calculations, and which would be retroactive to last year or perhaps more.

[2]Reprint of an article by Dena Seiden, who teaches ethics of health care organization at Columbia University's School of Public Health. Reprinted by permission from *Commonweal*, 113: 8–10, 12–13. Ja 17 '86. Copyright © 1986 by Commonweal Foundation.

There is a welter of anecdotal evidence and soft data regarding malpractice. The lack of hard data has a variety of causes: the expense of a major study, the uncertainty about whose interest it serves to fund such a study, and the difficulty in deciding what to measure, whether equity issues, improvement of physician performance, effect on community health and finances, or other possible factors. Nonetheless, the increasing resort to malpractice suits and the growing size of the settlements can be documented. The 40 percent rise in the number of physicians practicing from 1960 to 1978 may account in part for the 24 percent rise in frequency of claims in the same time period, and something similar may be happening currently. But the rise in the incidence of suit from 3.3 per 100 physicians prior to 1978 to 8.9 per 100 now demolish that as anything close to a full answer.

Data from New York show not only a 59.8 percent increase in the number of malpractice claims in that state between 1976 and 1983, but a 232 percent increase in the average size of the settlements, and a 556 percent (!) increase in the total cost of claims paid.

Certain specialties—neurosurgery, orthopedics, and obstetrics—have been particularly hard hit by the rise in suits. In New Jersey, for example, 60 percent of obstetricians have been sued more than once. In New York, nearly 50 percent have been sued three or more times. Why the astounding amount of litigation in obstetrics? Speculation has centered on at least four reasons: the current expectation of having a normal if not a perfect child, an expectation heightened if couples have fewer children and focus greater hopes on those they do have; the depersonalization in obstetrician/patient relationships resulting when the doctor for pre-natal care may not be the delivering doctor; the increase in the number of handicapped babies who survive infancy because of improved technology but then need long-term, very expensive care; and the new technologies themselves, which open up whole new areas of controversy.

Whatever the reasons for increased litigation, physicians are reacting strongly. For the last two years, virtually every professional medical journal and the bulletins of nearly every state medical society have been replete with articles reflecting the belief that physicians are beleaguered by a hostile society and battered by fee-crazed lawyers, and consequently are adopting defensive postures to deal with the potential of suit. A key issue is, in fact, the extent to which the increased threat of suit is influencing physicians' behavior. Are they ordering unnecessary tests and procedures, refusing to handle certain types of cases or perform other procedures, leaving areas where malpractice insurance rates and incidence of suit are high, or even stopping practice entirely?

Relocating or abandoning a medical practice is obviously a drastic—but evidently increasingly thinkable—response to the malpractice threat. These are figures from the Medical Society of New York:

A Comparison of Three Surveys in Which New York-trained Resident Physicians Were Asked Whether They Would Stay in New York or Relocate Out-of-State

	1980	1983	1985
Will Practice Medicine in New York	87%	69%	46%
Will Relocate Out-of-State	13%	27%	42%
Undecided		4%	12%

Such findings support the impression that physicians, especially those just leaving residencies, are increasingly willing to pack their bags and move to states like Indiana where high malpractice premiums and frequent suits do not occur, in part because of tough state laws controlling the nature and amounts of suit. Indiana has a $1,200 average premium, South Dakota a $1,500 average. Ohio, a more urbanized industrial state, has an average of $4,000, compared with New York's average of $16,500. In 1984, New York premiums rose to $53,676 for obstetricians and $63,311 for neurosurgeons.

It is possible to argue that this represents, at long last, a way of redistributing the physician surplus to better serve medically needy areas. Such a redistribution, however, is by definition unplanned, and may simply result in a glut of physicians in new areas, and a dearth in others. Or certain types of services may simply become unavailable in some localities. Dr. Charles Gibbs of the American College of Obstetrics/Gynecology Commission of Professional Liability says that many obstetricians are giving up their practices, particularly those with high-risk patients. Patients will have to find care in "expensive, sometimes distant health centers, or from less qualified providers."

The shift from one geographical area to others is paralleled by the shift from one form of medical organization to others. Physicians are more and more seeking salaried posts in a variety of institutions: the profit-making hospital chains, health maintenance organizations (HMOs), medical schools, and teaching hospitals. Malpractice is only one of many causes for this shift. But malpractice insurance and legal counsel are fringe benefits of these jobs and may be encouraging the change in the physician's role from individual entrepreneur to company employee. The outcome for medical practice is likely to be a kind of standardization in care. That may sometimes mean a greater evenness in quality but with some risk to likelihood of innovations. For once an overall treatment protocol is established, any deviation in favor of a new method may be perceived as potential grounds for lawsuit.

Some patients and some physicians may be dramatically affected by the pressure to relocate or abandon medical practice, or to take up salaried positions. Affecting even more patients and physicians—and indeed everyone paying taxes or insurance premiums—is the resort to "defensive medicine," i.e., measures physicians use to protect themselves against suits. In 1973 the Department of Health, Education, and Welfare attempted a definitive study of the malpractice issue and concluded that the extent to which defensive medicine was practiced was not then known. A 1984 study from the Harvard School of Public Health predicts that in 1986 the costs of defensive medicine will total $42 billion from "unnecessary invasion diagnostic procedures, excessive medical testing, and unneeded days of hospitalization." The American Medical Association estimates that defensive medicine added $15.1 billion to the cost of American medical care in 1983, and such practices are assumed by the profession to account for 30–40 percent of all diagnostic procedures.

An American College of Obstetrics/Gynecology survey shows 55 percent of its membership are abstaining from high risk deliveries because of fear of malpractice suits, and 18 percent are abandoning all obstetrical practice. The same survey showed obstetricians and gynecologists are:

• becoming more selective about their patients; and referring patients to other physicians more frequently;

• performing less gynecological surgery and more diagnostic tests, passing those costs on to patients and/or third-party payers;

- obtaining written consent more often;
- providing written or taped information to patients more frequently;
- increasingly having other staff present at examinations;
- increasing fees by 10 percent and more over the last two years to cover the higher malpractice premiums (in New York State, 50 percent of obstetricians and gynecologists have increased their fees by 20 percent or more over the last two years).

This is clearly a mixed bag of items; some, such as "written consent" and "more information to the patient," tend to improve patient care. Some factors are more complex: more frequent referrals, for example, are not simply to garner second opinions, many of which are merely protective, but are often an attempt to drop "high-risk" patients. The underlying question is: to what degree are these changes predicated on a fear of suit rather than on the trend in the last two decades toward greater public awareness of patient rights, health education, etc., and the simultaneous diminishing of physician autonomy? The negative side of defensive medicine is difficult to attribute to any cause other than fear of suit. It is highly damaging to anything other than the most conservative patient care. It affects physician-patient relationships, pitting one against the other as potential adversaries. It undermines attempts to contain health care costs.

Consider the question of rising rates of birth by Caesarean section. The Medical Society of New Jersey journal notes that while in 1984 the rate of Caesarean section was one in five, in the Northeast it is one in three or two in five. There is speculation that some of this is the result of improved anesthetic techniques, new antibiotics, technological development in electronic fetal monitoring, the age of the population presently giving birth, and the old adage, once a Caesarean, always a Caesarean. But obstetricians' fear of malpractice suits is cited as an overriding reason. In a borderline case, the possible damages of not doing a Caesarean outweigh the risks of doing one. The Harvard School of Public Health study mentioned above predicts 200,000 Caesarean sections a year which are not medically indicated, but done for fear of suit because vaginal birth might be claimed to have damaged an infant.

Statistics like these much be complemented by a close look at individual cases. Physicians are appalled, of course, when a single award in Florida for an obstetric case was $12,500,000. Or when a jury awarded $83,037 to a fourteen-year-old boy whose surgeon had removed too much of a chronic ingrown toenail and cauterized the root so it couldn't grow back.

But the real ethical difficulties can only be recognized when a problem like borderline Caesareans is seen in terms of a frequently cited case, *Trotman vs. New York Hospital*, New York Supreme Court, No. 9175/77, June 22, 1983. Here the jury "awarded $3,318,000 to the plaintiff whose new-born male infant suffers from mild cerebral palsy as a result of traumatic vaginal delivery." The award is staggering, though one would want to know the definition of a "mild" palsy. However, the case history states that the resident physician found the infant in a breech position and did not report it. Further, that the child was still appearing in a reverse of the normal head-first position, that is, feet first with one foot caught behind his head, when the mother's membrane spontaneously ruptured five hours later. Diagnostic x-ray pelvimetry, which in a case like this would be standard medical practice, was not performed.

Cases like this make malpractice the inflammatory issue it is for both sides. The award was of such magnitude that it has led to a precipitous rise in premium rates and significantly inflated the cost of care for the community as a whole. But the negligence of the physicians was so clearly manifest that it cried out for redress.

Consider the case of *Unana vs. Torrance Memorial Hospital*, Los Angeles Superior Court, No. 22-681, December, 1982. The patient plaintiff had been admitted in active labor, with a chart noting previous fetal heart irregularities. This was confirmed by fetal monitoring one hour after admission. The obstetrical resident notified the attending physician one hour after that. The attending physician did not arrive. Four hours after admission, fetal distress was again monitored, and the resident again reported the information to the obstetrician by phone. The attending physician arrived two hours after the second call. A Caesarean section was done, but the child had suffered brain injury with severe mental and motor retardation. The award in the case was $1 million.

Taking note of these cases is not an attempt to prove that physicians are fatally flawed, wildly negligent, uninformed, and uncaring members of society. It *is* an attempt to prove what both society and physicians seem to be invested in forgetting: physicians are members of the same fallen, finite human species as the rest of us, and as such, can do great harm, as can we all.

Such harm falls first, and most immediately, on individuals

who should be able to protect themselves against injury and negligence. But the needs and rights of these specific, identifiable, gravely injured individuals must be seen in relation to the needs and rights of the community—that is, of a larger number of unidentifiable individuals who may suffer the less grave but more widespread burden of higher costs, unnecessary procedures, or inaccessible care.

Our present system of malpractice litigation has at least two major purposes, and one can argue that neither of them is being served well.

The first purpose is essentially retrospective—providing redress for individuals and families who have been seriously and negligently injured. The 1973 H.E.W. study mentioned above indicates that this is a real problem. In an appendix to that report, H.E.W. estimated that physician-caused injuries may constitute 7.5 percent of general medical and gynecological cases—but also that remarkably few of these negligence cases result in suits. So many factors apparently determine who does or does not undertake litigation and what the eventual outcome is that, for purposes of redressing injury, the malpractice system seems more like a lottery than a reliable source of patient protection.

The way the malpractice system operates also forces us to reflect on the exact nature of "redress." The legal code which Moses gave to the tribes of Israel—e.g., "an eye for an eye and a tooth for a tooth"—is sometimes presented as barbaric, but it was, in truth, actually meant to both soften and democratize the previous Near-Eastern codes. These allowed *more* than equal compensation—the death penalty, say, for the wrongful destruction of an eye. They also meted out penalties on a class basis. Loss of an aristocrat's eye might merit the death penalty; a commoner's eye might cost another eye; a slave's eye, merely a payment of money. In these terms, our present malpractice compensation system is, if anything, pre-Mosaic. Instead of a distinctly reciprocal amount of compensation for a given injury, it adds on an award for the vague category "pain and suffering." Juries can award no amount, a minimal amount, or a huge amount for the same medical injury, depending on an individual jury's make-up and predilections. This catch-as-catch-can system compares to the inequitable results of pre-Mosaic law codes, rather than a more equitable loss-for-loss approach. The expense incurred to raise a badly damaged child must be provided parents who choose not to make such a child a ward of the state. Malpractice settlements are one, although not necessarily the best, way of doing that. Other ways include direct government subsidies to the parents, tax deductions or credits, expanded and improved systems of free child care and education. But none of this is really compensation for the injury itself—a notion that is actually fairly repulsive. "Pain and suffering" money will not restore the child's well-being, nor give the parents the joy of raising a normal, healthy child. It is not surprising that eliminating or restricting the "pain and suffering" category is one of the staples of recent proposals for malpractice reform.

Reform is all the more obviously needed when one looks at a second major purpose the malpractice system is supposed to be serving. This is essentially a *prospective* purpose, namely to deter physicians, through the threat of punishment, from negligently harming patients in the future. This second rationale behind malpractice suits, in other words, is to force physicians into becoming better physicians while dealing with those who practice bad medicine. There is little evidence, beyond that cited earlier regarding defensive medicine, that this has happened. In many ways, defensive medicine is worse medicine. The threat of malpractice lowers rather than raises the quality of physician performance. And it is the public, both as taxpayers and as medical patients, who largely end up bearing the burden of that "punishment" meant to discipline physicians. The cost of malpractice premiums is passed on to the public; the cost of unnecessary procedures becomes part of the national health bill. If defensive medicine is only half as widely practiced as current estimates would have it, if only 20 percent of our diagnostic tests are unnecessary, or if only $21 billion is being uselessly spent, those still represent huge losses, particularly at a time of retrenchment in health care expenditures.

When it comes to improving physician practice, more direct methods—education and professional peer assessment—are much more likely to succeed than the massive deterrence of malpractice penalties. Better physicians are apt to be created through different types of medical school programs or different admissions standards, by monitoring and acting on consistently poor physician performance through state medical societies and state licensing agencies, or by rapidly removing impaired physicians from patient contact and getting them into treatment. Malpractice litigation, by contrast, can scarcely be an incentive for closer professional scrutiny. It is rather an occasion for circling the professional wagons.

Caught between active professional constituencies, (physicians and lawyers, as well as health consumer groups and specialized lobbies such as the American Association of Retired People), government officials have been reluctant to make any bold moves. The Gephardt-Moore bill, sponsored by Richard A. Gephardt (D-Mo.) and W. Henson Moore (R-La.), has been introduced in Congress for the second time. It proposes a number of serious reforms, though for federal health programs only, and is given little chance of serious consideration, much less passage. Its most controversial sections would limit awards to economic loss (medical bills, rehabilitation fees, loss of work income, attorneys' costs), and eliminate awards for "pain and suffering," punitive damages, and other general damages. Though some states (notably California, whose Supreme Court in March 1985 upheld a $250,000 cap on "pain and suffering") have limited noneconomic loss awards, none has done so as radically as the Gephardt-Moore proposal. The bill would also offer compensation within six months and let settlements with a loss of over $5,000 be determined by a competent court.

New York State passed a more modest bill last June as an interim measure while a fuller solution was under study. Its major features are a mélange of limitations on lawyers' contingency fees (alleged by physicians to be the stick that whips the legal profession into a frenzy of malpractice litigation); pre-trial disclosure of expert witnesses; a mandatory *offer* of arbitration, which the patient would have the right to refuse; future periodic instead of lump-sum payments for awards over $1,000; and imposition of legal costs for frivolous suits. The *New York Times* editorially criticized this interim bill as insufficient, particularly for not limiting awards for "pain and suffering." In a special session last December, the New York legislature failed to pass any further legislation on the subject. That meant that the interim measure's freeze on malpractice premiums was no longer in effect, and one insurance carrier has already applied for a 76 percent increase in rates.

Other solutions have been proposed. In 1978, the Institute of Medicine, the medical section of the National Academy of Sciences, published a study of six alternative systems:

- traditional litigation—the present system;
- pre-trial screening panels—using peer and/or lay review boards to try to halt frivolous suits, suits in which one party is

likely to concede, and so on, so as to reduce the burden on the courts and facilitate speedy trials;

• arbitration—again, peer and/or lay review boards working outside the court system to resolve the substantive issues in malpractice claims;

• medical adversity insurance—automatic compensation for injury, to be financed by physicians in some pooling method, with compensation determined by a pre-fixed schedule;

• elective no-fault—use of the same principles currently operating with auto insurance to provide coverage which patients could voluntarily choose, with the further option of court suit;

• social insurance—similar to medical adversity insurance, but publicly financed.

The Institute evaluated these systems by various criteria, from cost to deterrence of injury. It looked for fairness both for injured patients and for providers. With much hesitation it came down in favor of arbitration.

Around the same time Clark C. Havighurst argued persuasively in the *Duke Law Journal* for medical adversity insurance. Injuries would be automatically compensated; the amount of the compensation would be pre-established according to the type of injury. Compensation for injuries not listed could be adjudicated, but it is assumed that the list of "relatively avoidable" medical injuries would be fairly comprehensive. This alternative would remove the threat of outsized (and, in any case, unpredictable) awards. The hooker, of course, is the total expense of the proposal, given the large number of "routine" medical consequences arising in the course of treatment and hospitalization—most of them *not* currently resulting in compensation.

There may be no perfectly satisfactory alternative to our current malpractice system, but at least part of a solution is at hand. It would include the limitation of malpractice awards to the actual economic burden incurred by injured parties. The Association of Trial Lawyers of America asks, "What is fair compensation for the permanent loss of the use of a child's brain? How do you determine the damages for the permanent loss of sight? How do you compensate for a permanent inability to walk?" The questions are meant to be rhetorical, to oppose limits on awards. Actually, they point in the opposite direction. There can be *no* compensation for permanent loss of a child's brain, for blindness, crippling, etc., per se. What can be determined—although still not without difficulty—is the economic costs of the injury, and that can constitute the settlement. If the cause was negligence, and punitive measures are in order, or if other patients need to be protected, then the physician's license to practice should be limited or removed. If the cause turns out to be, as best we can tell in our present state of knowledge, an unavoidable risk of modern medicine, then there is only the knowledge, many millennia old, that life is tragic and humankind flawed. Penalizing the full community financially, and affecting both its access to care and the quality of its care, in order to deal with the tragedies of some individuals and the failings of others, is neither equitable nor just. Limiting malpractice damages to actual economic costs would be both ethical and practically significant: New York State's largest malpractice insurer, Medical Liability Mutual Insurance Company, reports that the component of "pain and suffering" in all jury verdicts from January 1980 through June 1985 was no less than 55.1 percent of the total awards. In the nine states with a $250,000 cap on awards, average premiums range from 7 percent to 42 percent of the New York State average.

The present system has very little ethical ground on which to stand, other than vengeance, a motive society might want to diminish rather than foster. Careful investigation of alternatives, such as arbitration, social insurance, and medical adversity insurance, should be undertaken before the whole system collapses, and before—in what has now become the typical American approach to health care—we jerrybuild another reform on sand, not rock, and watch it sink in the next storm.

MED SCHOOLS LEARN HUMILITY[3]

In 1985 David Schrader was a biology major at Johns Hopkins, planning to go to medical school. Then he reconsidered the costly and grueling 10 years ahead of him—and headed for law instead. Schrader is not alone: applications to medical schools have dropped 26 percent since 1975, and early projections for the

[3]Reprint of an article by *Newsweek* staff writer James N. Baker. Reprinted by permission from *Newsweek*, 109: 61–62. Je 29 '87. Copyright © 1987 Newsweek Inc.

entering class of 1987 are off another 10 percent. The ratio of applicants to places has gone from 3 to 1 in the mid-1970s to less than 2 to 1 today, and students who do apply have lower grade-point averages. "We may be getting down to the threshold of quality," warns Dr. August Swanson of the Association of American Medical Colleges. The drop-off at dental schools has been staggering—63 percent over the past decade. In the spring of 1987 Georgetown University announced that it would close its dental school, the nation's second largest, in 1990.

School administrators blame the drop in applications on everything from fear of AIDS to "me"-generation values. Students once attracted to medicine in part for its lucrative salaries now find they can get rich faster in business or investment banking—while working shorter hours and racking up far less debt; these days, the average med student graduates owing more than $33,000—and debt loads more than twice that amount are not uncommon. Fear of malpractice suits and rising insurance costs are also discouraging students, just when cost-containment measures and the trend toward group medical care have diminished the field's prestige. "The loss of autonomy and drop in salaries," says Schrader, "make medicine not worth it."

The prognosis is not necessarily negative for the profession. Dental and medical schools boomed in the 1970s, creating a glut of dentists and an expected surplus of doctors by 1990. The diminished competition may help attract a different breed of student. "It's good," says University of Illinois student Marc Nudelman, "if it takes the purely-for-profit people out of the pool." The biggest decline has been in applications from white males, creating more room for women and minorities. Now that schools no longer have their pick of grinds with 4.0 grade averages, "anybody with over a 3.0 should consider it—especially if he has other attributes," says the American Medical Association's Dr. John Tupper.

Still, some schools are reducing class sizes rather than lowering admissions standards. Howard University just cut its incoming class from 128 to an even 100. Emory and Oral Roberts universities have also eliminated dental programs. Other institutions—including prestigious Johns Hopkins—are considering marketing campaigns, and some plan to recruit high schoolers before they are irretrievably committed to computers. "No doubt we'll even have to go into grade schools," says Dr. Donald Hare of the University of Rochester.

'The Same Fishbowl'

In particular, experts believe that schools could do more to recruit minority students. Asian-American applicants have doubled in the last decade—and women now make up nearly a third of the pool. "If they hadn't increased," says Swanson, "we'd have been in big trouble before now." But blacks and Hispanics remain underrepresented. Medical student Garfield Bryant, who is black, was personally called by the admissions dean of the University of Michigan, which reports a 40 percent increase in qualified minority applicants since 1978. But not every school has made such efforts. "The problem," says Dr. C. M. Scott of the University of Alabama, "is that all the schools fish in the same fishbowl." Dr. Frederick Greene of George Washington University believes that money is to blame: "It's difficult for a kid from a poor background to accept a loan equal to his family's income."

Vigorous recruiting and financial-aid programs may both be needed in the next decade if the surplus starts to dwindle. Early retirement by disgruntled older practitioners and long leaves by women with families could easily confound the numbers. And there are still spot shortages of doctors and dentists in inner cities and rural areas, which the smaller classes will no doubt accentuate. One thing is certain: scrambling for students has been a humbling experience for medical and dental schools. What Dr. James Taren of the University of Michigan describes as their "patrician attitude" has gone the way of the house call on Sunday afternoon.

FED UP, FEARFUL AND FRAZZLED[4]

December 1986. New York City. A patient at Montefiore Medical Center could have died when his tracheal breathing tube fell out. Reason: no one on the understaffed night shift heard the respirator alarm go off.

February 1987. Los Angeles. Six days after being released from the Los Angeles County University of Southern California

[4]Reprint of an article by *Time* staff writer Christine Gorman. Reprinted by permission from *Time*, 131: 77–78. Nov 14 '89. Copyright © 1988 Time Inc.

Medical Center, a 39-year-old woman dies from complications suffered in a hospital-bed fire. Her family's contention: harried nurses discovered the accident only after she had suffered burns on 40% of her body.

January 1988. Louisville. For a time, by astonishing coincidence, none of the city's eleven hospitals can accept critically ill or injured patients. Reason: available beds in intensive-care units cannot be filled because not enough nurses are on duty.

From New York to Los Angeles, the nation's hospitals are locked in the grip of what could become the worst nursing shortage since World War II. Overworked and abysmally paid, growing numbers of America's 2 million registered nurses, 97% of whom are women, are trading in their bedpans for law books, ledgers and briefcases. The exodus of the exhausted comes at a time when nursing schools are reporting dramatic declines in enrollment and veteran nurses are loudly objecting to their working conditions. Paradoxically, however, there are more nurses employed now than ever before. Thanks to increasingly complex medical technology, an aging patient population and the worsening AIDS epidemic, the demand for nurses has never been greater.

Alarmed by gathering signs of a health-care disaster, Secretary of Health and Human Services Otis Bowen recently convened a special commission in Washington to find ways to revitalize the nursing profession. Almost simultaneously, retired Admiral James Watkins, the chairman of the presidential AIDS panel, called for federal programs to attract half a million more nurses by 1991 to treat AIDS patients and others who are chronically ill. Nurses on the job bluntly admit that patients entering U.S. hospitals these days may be risking their lives. "You should be worried if you or someone in your family has to check into a hospital," warns Mary Helen Clark, an intensive-care nurse at Einstein-Weiler Hospital in the Bronx. "There is not enough staffing to cover shifts. Patient care is compromised all the time."

In desperation, nurses have taken to the streets to protest. In January, 3,200 nurses staged a 3½ day strike against the Los Angeles County public-hospital system. Hospitals in the New York City area have endured two strikes and four sickouts in the past eight weeks alone. "You have to be deaf, dumb and blind not to know that there's a dangerous situation," says Emergency Room Nurse Renee Gestone, who picketed Brooklyn's Lutheran Medical Center last week. Adds fellow Striker Pat Stewart: "Some of the doctors are saying that we are morally wrong to go on strike, but is it any more morally wrong than if we are stretched out thin, giving bad care?"

"Who wants to go into nursing these days when there are so many better opportunities for women?" asks Adriene Barmann, 27, a cancer nurse at Mount Sinai Medical Center in Miami Beach. For most registered nurses, the average beginning salary is $21,000, yet 30-year veterans regularly earn less than $30,000. Duties range from starting intravenous lines and bathing patients to such menial tasks as fixing TVs and taking out the garbage. Hospitals routinely require 50- and 60-hour workweeks. Little wonder, then, that enrollment in nursing schools has plummeted 20%, to less than 200,000 student nurses, since 1983. During that period, four of the nation's top nursing schools have closed their doors.

At the same time, advances in medical technology have dramatically increased nurses' responsibilities. Consider the neurological intensive-care unit of Chicago's Cook County Hospital. Cocooned in a bewildering array of intravenous lines, tubes and machines, each patient is desperately ill; 30 nurses are required to monitor and care properly for a group of nine patients around the clock. "Things can change rapidly," explains Mary O'Flaherty, the unit's nurse coordinator. "One moment a patient's intracranial pressures, blood pressure and cerebral-profusion pressure can be fine. The next moment you can start hearing bells."

Patients now require more attention outside the intensive-care unit as well. As part of a long overdue campaign to control soaring medical costs, most patients are released from the hospital faster, but the ones who remain are sicker—and usually older. The number of elderly patients has almost doubled in the past two decades. Result: more nurses are needed for fewer patients.

The AIDS epidemic has only made a bad situation worse. In New York City, AIDS patients already take up 9% of all available hospital beds. "Caring for AIDS patients is different from caring for any other sick person, make no mistake," says Donna Stidham, a senior nurse at the 20-bed AIDS unit of Sherman Oaks Community Hospital in Los Angeles. These patients tend to be sicker, their illnesses less predictable and their families more difficult to handle. Experimental treatments require close attention and study. "It's going to make everyone face the nursing shortage," says Jeanne Kalinoski, an AIDS nurse at a major New York City hospital. "If you have a heart attack in the emergency room, you might not get a bed because of the number of AIDS patients."

Officially, of course, the shortage has not really endangered people's lives. "Often the level of T.L.C. that a patient expects—the back rub, the hand holding—doesn't get done in today's intense environment," says Allan Anderson, president of Lenox Hill Hospital in Manhattan. "But I don't think there is any evidence that the quality of hospital care has deteriorated."

Nurses tell more troubling tales. Some are required to "float" into sections of the hospital where they have no experience; others must work beyond the point of exhaustion with no backup. Cook County Hospital's O'Flaherty contends that it is not at all unusual for a nurse to be confronted with two patients requiring emergency attention at the same time. Once on the scene, of course, nurses are legally liable; they cannot refuse to work, however impossible the situation. The only recourse for many is to fill out a form protesting the assignment. This does not absolve them if something goes wrong, but it proves that the hospital knew about the situation. "Someone in the hospital fills out a form every night," says Einstein-Weiler's Clark.

What is the solution? Trying to attract young nurses by offering higher starting salaries is a first step. But the cost of constantly having to train new nurses drains the resources of virtually every major medical center. The money might be better spent on creating incentives for experienced nurses to stay. "Nurses who are competent and show potential for professional growth ought to be able to double their salaries in ten years and triple them by retirement," argues Judith Ryan, executive director of the American Nurses' Association, based in Kansas City. "That would make us competitive with other professions."

Many health-care experts believe the entire concept of nursing and the traditional role of the nurse must be radically redefined. For too long the medical community has depended on nurses as a source of cheap but versatile labor. "We need to define the professional nature of nurses more precisely and assign other people to positions where a nurse's professional and scientific background is not essential," says Dr. David Skinner, president of New York Hospital. It does not take a nursing degree, for example, to deliver a pill to a patient. Houston's M.D. Anderson Hospital sometimes uses medication technicians, not R.N.s [registered nurses] to dispense drugs to patients after nurses have verified the dose. Says Connie Curran, vice president for health-care management and patient services at the American Hospital Association (AHA) in Chicago: "Hospitals that are using registered nurses to answer telephones and do an incredible amount of paper work should hire a secretary and uses nurses to nurse."

Naturally, such a revamped job description means more responsibility—and more respect. Nurses are often the first to spot trouble, make sense of a patient's confusing symptoms or suggest a needed change in treatment. Yet acting on such observations has traditionally been the physician's purview. R.N.s must become full-fledged members of the team and be expected to engage in the medical give-and-take about patients' well-being. That role is never in doubt on the AIDS ward at Sherman Oaks Community Hospital, where doctors and nurses find themselves depending on one another to battle the deadly disease. Beth Israel Hospital in Boston has retained its reputation for first-rate care with an innovative program that gives each nurse primary responsibility for one or two patients.

Even so, nurses are not quite blameless in this crisis. If they want to be taken seriously in an era of high-tech medicine, they are going to have to get serious about educational norms and standardize training programs. Currently, students can choose to take an R.N. exam after completing courses that last from two to five years. And the pressure is on to expand less rigorous programs in order to produce more nurses. Says Paula Castonguay, a nurse recruiter at the University of Texas Medical Branch at Galveston: "It worries me that not only are we not going to have enough nurses, but the ones we get are going to be less qualified."

The medical community can no longer afford to chew up its nurses and spit them out. "The old attitude toward nurses—'work long, work late, work hard'—is just not going to attract people," says Debbie Davenport, a Los Angeles nurse. Agrees the AHA's Curran: "Nurses aren't content to be the housewives of the hospital anymore." Nor should they be.

HOSPITAL CARE FOR PROFIT[5]

In 1961, four men set our for a game of golf. Two were real estate agents; two, young lawyers from a prestigious Louisville,

[5]Reprint of an article by Geraldine Dallek, a health policy analyst at the National Health Law Program, a legal services support center specializing in legal health issues affecting the poor. Reprinted by permission from *Society*, 23:54–59. Jl/Ag '86. Copyright © 1986 by Transaction Publishers.

Kentucky, law firm. That golf game was the beginning of what was to become an international corporation with $2.6 billion in annual revenue—Humana, Incorporated. Only a few years later, in 1968, two Nashville doctors met with Jack Massey, a founder of Kentucky Fried Chicken, and Hospital Corporation of America (HCA), the nation's largest for-profit hospital chain, was born. By 1984, HCA owned or managed 260 hospitals in 41 states and grossed more than $3.9 billion from its hospitals and nursing homes. By the mid-1980s, proprietary hospitals controlled 12 percent of the acute care hospital market in the United States, 21 percent in the South.

It is possible to understand the rapid growth and impact of these proprietary chains only by examining the environment that nurtured them. In many ways, the medical care industry is like the defense industry. First, the goals of each—protecting our nation and protecting our health—are intrinsically valued by our society. Second, medical care and national defense are extremely costly. We spend $300 billion on defense each year, three-fourths as much as the $400 billion spent on health care. Third, both industries, in what is clearly aberrant free-market behavior, have been permitted to set the price of the goods and services they produce. In defense, it is the weapons contractors who have been virtually given a blank check; in the medical industry, hospitals, nursing homes, drug manufacturers, and physicians have, until very recently, also had carte blanche to determine how much their product is worth. Given these factors, is it any wonder that both industries are highly profitable?

The ability to make money from the delivery of medical care is not new. In the late nineteenth century, as hospitals became safe and attractive places in which to care for the ill, small for-profit hospitals sprung up in the United States and Western Europe. In Europe, individual for-profit hospitals faded from the scene as government assumed more responsibility for ensuring the provision of health care. By contrast, the for-profit hospital industry in the United States flourished.

In the early 1980s, for-profit chains were the darling of Wall Street with a 20 percent growth rate. During 1982, a recession year for most businesses, stocks of the top four hospital chains rose 30 percent. Profits of the twenty largest chains went up 38 percent in 1983 and 28.5 percent the following year. In 1984, HCA's chief executive officer was the second highest paid executive in the nation, and the head of National Medical Enterprises

(NME) beat out the movie moguls as the highest paid executive in Southern California.

What accounts for the rapid expansion and huge profits of these new hospital organizations? Traditional reimbursement policies go far to explain the attractiveness of the hospital industry to entrepreneurs. Hospitals, until adoption of the new Medicare diagnosis related group (DRG) payment system in 1983, were generally paid by a retrospective cost-based reimbursement system. This open-ended system for paying hospitals, begun by Blue Cross plans (acting almost as agents for the hospitals) after World War II, was adopted by the federal government as the quid pro quo for the hospital industry's support of Medicare and Medicaid legislation in 1965. The potential for profits in this reimbursement system cannot be overstated. "It was hard not to be successful," commented the chief executive officer of National Medical Enterprises in a 1985 *Wall Street Journal* article. Profits could be made by simply buying existing hospitals and making sure that bills to both private and public insurers contained an add-on profit.

Hospitals could be bought easily in the seventies and early eighties. For-profit chains' access to capital through the sale of stock gave them an advantage over their nonprofit brethren for purposes of both building and buying hospitals. Because of their large revenue, assets, and equity base, they were viewed as sound financial risks.

The major growth of for-profit chains came from the purchase of financially troubled hospitals. Between 1980 and 1982, 43 percent of the growth of the six largest for-profit chains came from the purchase of other for-profit hospitals, mostly independent facilities. A third of the growth came from the construction of new hospitals and a fourth from the purchase of public and voluntary nonprofit hospitals. Following a for-profit purchase, ailing hospitals were brought back to health by building new facilities to attract physicians, substantially increasing charges, and reducing services to those who could not pay. Public hospitals owned and run by local governments were often receptive to being bailed out by for-profit chains. Faced with aging facilities, unable to attract privately insured patients, and confronted with increased numbers of the poor seeking care, public hospitals awash with red ink were all too happy to sell to for-profit chains.

In assessing the impact of the for-profit hospital industry, we must go well beyond the counting of beds. The industry has had a far-reaching impact on the cost of hospital care, the delivery of services to the poor, and the behavior of other health care providers.

Costly Care

For-profit chains have often been viewed favorably because of their promise to bring managerial efficiency to the "wasteful" nonprofit sector. It does not appear that they possess superior managerial talents. After reviewing a number of studies on multi-hospital systems, Ermann and Gabel concluded in a May 1985 article in *Medical Care* that "There is little empirical evidence that [multihospital] systems have realized economies of scale of mass purchasing or use capital facilities more efficiently." Nor have chains served as a competitive catalyst to an industry grown fat by its insulation from free-market forces. Theoretically, competition and efficiency would lead to reduced costs. Judged by this standard, for-profit hospital chains also failed, as they increased, not lowered, the cost of hospital care.

For-profit chain costs have been higher than nonprofit hospital costs for three reasons: they mark up charges well above expenses; they use more expensive ancillary services than nonprofit facilities; and charges must cover their higher capital costs. According to several studies, the difference in costs between for-profit and not-for-profit hospitals is substantial. A comparison of charges at 280 California for-profit and nonprofit hospitals showed that for-profit hospital charges per admission were 24 percent higher than those of the voluntary hospitals and 47 percent higher than public hospital charges. According to this study—by Robert Pattison and Hallie Katz, reported in the August 1983 *New England Journal of Medicine*—huge profits were made in ancillary services such as pharmacy and laboratory services. The study also showed that despite the claims of administrative savings, costs for "fiscal services" and "administrative services" (which include costs to maintain corporate headquarters elsewhere) were 32 percent higher in for-profit chain hospitals than in voluntary hospitals. The authors concluded that the data "do not support the claim that investor-owned chains enjoy overall operating efficiencies or economies of scale in administrative fiscal services."

Results of a more recent study, by Lewin and Associates and health policy analysts at Johns Hopkins University, of eighty matched pairs of investor-owned chain and not-for-profit hospitals in eight states were remarkably similar to the Pattison and Katz study: prices charged by for-profit chain hospitals were 22 percent more per admission than those charged by matched not-for-profit hospitals.

For-profit hospitals also charge more for several procedures, according to a 1983 Blue Cross/Blue Shield of North Carolina study. Comparing charges for three commonly performed hospital procedures—gall bladder removals, hysterectomies, and normal deliveries of babies—at six for-profit hospitals and six matched nonprofit hospitals, the study found that in all but one case the average total charge was from 6 percent to 58 percent higher in the for-profit hospitals.

Patients have generally been insulated from higher for-profit charges by their third party coverage. Nevertheless, at least one Las Vegas man found the cost of care at his local for-profit hospital upsetting. In a June 1985 letter to the *Las Vegas Review Journal,* the gentleman recounted how he had

> recently had the misfortune of requiring emergency room treatment at Humana Sunrise Hospital for kidney stone problems. This was my second encounter with this problem. The first encounter occurred last July, and I was treated at Southern Nevada Memorial Hospital.
>
> As the treatment was almost identical, I have had the opportunity to compare the costs of the two facilities. I was not surprised to find that Humana hospitals were more expensive; however, I was shocked to discover that the cost was fully 50% above that of Southern Nevada.
>
> As I was curtly informed by administrative personnel at Humana, the costs were higher because Humana is a "private" hospital, and Southern Nevada is a county hospital. Now this is a point well taken and probably could account for a 15 or 20% difference, but 50%—Come on, who does Humana think they are fooling?

For-profit hospitals have also increased health care costs indirectly by building unneeded hospitals. For example, primarily because of the growth of for-profit hospitals, twelve Florida counties, underbedded in 1972, had 6,600 excess beds three years later. The for-profit chains that had controlled 16.7 percent of beds in 1972 had built 60 percent of the new beds.

If efficiency is measured by maximum use of the physical plant, for-profit chains are once again found wanting. In 1985, average hospital occupancy rates for the four largest proprietary chains ranged from 46 percent to 56 percent. Empty beds were not as important under the old cost-based reimbursement system, as charges to insurers for patients in the occupied beds could be increased to cover the cost of unoccupied beds. This changed with Medicare's new reimbursement system which pays a flat rate based on a patient's diagnosis and vigorous cost containment programs begun by Medicaid and private health insurers in 1983 and 1984.

The old cost-based reimbursement systems not only rewarded hospitals for providing extra services and hiking up prices but failed to penalize them for empty beds. Medicare's new flat rate reimbursement scheme provides opposite incentives: it rewards hospitals for reducing services (the fewer services provided, the more money made) and penalizes them for their empty beds. This dramatic change in the way hospitals are paid would, it could be supposed, hurt most those hospitals that had taken greatest advantage of the old system. This seems to have happened. In October of 1985, announcements by the leading chains of flat or reduced earnings stunned Wall Street and resulted in a steep decline in their stocks.

In response to changes in hospital reimbursement and declining hospital revenues, chains began to diversify—investing in more lucrative areas of medical care, including nursing homes, insurance companies, health maintenance organizations (HMOs), neighborhood emergicenters (often called doc-in-the-box), and home health agencies. Their proven ability to maximize profits from the provision of medical services will thus be tested in new arenas. Called a "managed system" approach, this vertical integration of the health industry gives proprietary chains added power to shape the future of health care delivery in this country.

Analysts may argue over the exact impact of the growth of the proprietary chains, but most agree that in subtle and not-so-subtle ways chains have irrevocably changed the milieu in which hospitals operate. Nowhere has the change been more profound than in the provision of hospital care to the poor.

Turning Away the Poor

Chains make no secret of their view that health care is nothing more than an economic commodity to be sold in the marketplace for a profit. One Humana senior vice president put it this way: "health care is a necessity, but so is food. Do you know of any neighborhood grocery store where you can walk out with $3,000 worth of food that you haven't paid for?" Chain spokesmen are also commonly heard to claim that their hospitals' commitment to the poor is taken care of by the payment of taxes. Given this view, it is not surprising that several state studies have found large disparities in the amount of care for the indigent provided by for-profit hospitals and voluntary and public hospitals. Typically, public hospitals provide the lion's share of uncompensated care; voluntary hospitals come in a poor second, with for-profit facilities running a dismal third.

Although for-profit hospitals constituted 32 percent of Florida's hospitals in 1983, they provided only 4 percent of the net charity care provided within the state. Florida's Hospital Cost Containment Board openly criticized for-profit hospitals in its 1983–84 annual report for their failure to share the burden of serving the uninsured poor. According to a report by the Texas Task Force on Indigent Health Care, for-profit hospitals made up 19.1 percent of the hospitals in that state in 1983, but provided less than 1 percent of the charity care and only 2.7 percent of the bad debt. Nonprofit hospitals, while making up 36.1 percent of the hospital facilities in Texas, provided 13.1 percent of charity care and 42.8 percent of the bad debt. Texas's public facilities provided most of the care of the poor: public hospitals, constituting 44.7 percent of the hospitals in the state, provide 86.9 percent of the charity care and 54.6 percent of the bad debt.

Some national data on provision of care for the indigent are available from the January 1981 Office of Civil Rights (OCR) survey of all general, short-term hospitals in the United States. An analysis of OCR data on inpatient admitting practices showed that 9.5 percent of all hospital patients were uninsured in 1981; yet only 6 percent of patients treated at for-profit hospitals were uninsured while 16.8 percent of those treated at hospitals owned by state and local governments were uninsured. Alan Sager also used OCR data in his study of hospital closures and relocation in 52 cities. He found that of the 4,038 patients categorized on admission as charity care patients (not to be charged) during the OCR survey, only 1 received care at a for-profit facility.

To some extent, the amount of charity care provided by for-profit hospitals is limited by their locations—in suburban white communities where few of the poor reside. When those hospitals are matched with similarly located nonprofit facilities, the amount of care to the poor differs little by ownership. However, geography does not explain why chain hospitals located in areas with significant numbers of uninsured populations provide so little in the way of charity.

The plight of one fifty-six-year-old uninsured laborer described in a recent *Washington Post* article is a case in point. Mr. G.R. Lafon sought care for third-degree grease burns on his side and back at the hospital nearest his home, a for-profit facility. The hospital and two other for-profit hospitals refused him emergency care because he did not have a deposit ranging from $500 to $1,500. One of the hospitals did take the precaution of inserting an intravenous tube and a catheter to stabilize his liquids before sending him on his way. After seven hours and a seventy-mile trek, Lafon arrived at Parkland Memorial Hospital in Dallas, the city's public hospital, where he was immediately admitted. Lafon required nineteen days of hospitalization and a skin graft for a cost of $22,000. Soon after discharge, he began receiving notices for an overdue hospital bill—not for the $22,000 owed to Parkland (that will be written off because Lafon is poor and uninsured) but for $373.75 from the for-profit facility to cover the cost of the catheter and intravenous tube.

Similar horror stories can be heard all over the South. In Memphis, for example, the city's largest HCA hospital threatened early in 1985 that it would stop chemotherapy treatments for a farmer with lung cancer when his family ran out of cash to continue his treatments. It was not until the day a suit was to be filed against the hospital claiming abandonment, denial of emergency medical care, intentional infliction of mental distress and extortion, that the HCA relented and agreed to continue treatment.

Voluntary hospitals and even some public hospitals also turn away the poor. What distinguishes the actions of for-profit chain hospitals from those of individual voluntary or public facilities is that the for-profit hospitals' policy of denying access is established at corporate headquarters and affects all their facilities throughout the nation. Although many voluntary hospitals are reducing their uncompensated care load in order to survive, others continue to view care for the poor as part of their mission.

The impact of care to the uninsured goes beyond the number of poor that proprietary chains do and do not serve. In the past five years, 180 public hospitals have been bought or managed by for-profit companies. This has resulted in an inexorable diminution of care to the poor: public officials do not sell hospitals in order to continue providing indigent care; they do so in order to relieve themselves from what they perceive as an onerous burden.

These sales, in turn, add to the financial troubles of the public and voluntary hospitals which continue to serve the indigent population. Chains also have had one other far-reaching effect on the provision of care to the poor: they have caused what Louanne Kennedy of the City University of New York describes as "the proprietarization of voluntary hospitals."

Beat 'Em or Join 'Em

Nonprofit hospitals have long had a split personality, torn by the need to make money (their business side) and the need to succor the poor and sick (their humanitarian or social side). The rapid growth of for-profit chains forced nonprofit facilities to come to terms with this dichotomy. In the process, hospitals became more businesslike and less concerned with humanitarian goals.

Interestingly, for-profit chains did promote competition in the delivery of hospital services but not, as the supply/demand curve predicts, on the basis of price. In the middle and late seventies, as the number of empty beds increased, hospital survival became increasingly predicated on attracting physicians who would admit their privately insured patients. In the competition for doctors, a hospital belonging to a large chain with easy access to capital had distinct advantages over the local voluntary and especially the public facility. A choice between a thirty-year-old public hospital with its leaky roof, overcrowded emergency room (filled with poor people), and frequent equipment breakdowns and the spanking new Humana or HCA hospital with the latest in diagnostic equipment and nary a poor person in sight, was no choice at all.

Chains also had the money to recruit doctors to their hospitals. For example, an April 5, 1982, Humana recruiting letter to pediatricians offered the following inducements to join a five-physician multispecialty group in Springhill, Louisiana:

> guaranteed income—$5,500 per month for the first six months; the lowest projected first-year income is $150,000;
> rent-free office—absolutely no business or other overhead expenses the first year; this includes a paid nurse, secretarial and office equipment and furniture, free utilities, and more;
> paid health/dental/life/malpractice insurance; company car; paid moving expenses; paid country club membership; paid on-site visit.

The most famous for-profit hospital recruit, Dr. William DeVries, was brought to the Humana Heart Institute in Louisville, Kentucky, with the promise of 100 artificial heart transplants.

In the competition over physicians, chains did not ignore the patient. Although price was not a consideration, well-heeled patients were lured to specialized chain facilities which touted the latest in sports medicine, treatment of diet disorders, wine and candlelight dinners for new parents, and a free hairstyle with a "tummy tuck." If patients were to be appealed to directly, then chain products had to be merchandized, and so advertising budgets became part and parcel of the cost of providing medical care.

At the same time as voluntary hospitals were losing private, paying patients to the new hospital on the block, they were also getting less money for the private, paying patients still filling their beds. Generally, under the blank-check reimbursement system, hospitals simply passed on the costs of their nonpaying patients to their privately insured patients whose care was paid for through employer-subsidized insurance. Thus, employers were subsidizing care for the poor through higher insurance premiums. While hospital access for the poor has been far from universal, a great deal of service was paid for by this cost shift. The health insurance industry estimated that it was charged an extra $8 billion in 1983 to subsidize the provision of care to those who could not pay and were uninsured.

As hospital costs kept spiraling (in some years by 20 percent) and as the number of uninsured poor increased, commercial insurors and business interests became less willing to pay this cost shift or what they called a "sick tax." Arguing that they should only have to pay premium costs to cover care for their work force, not the nation's poor, employers demanded and got reductions in their premium costs and the beginnings of competition based on price.

Voluntary and public hospitals subsidizing the poor are at a distinct disadvantage in any game based on price competition because they are, according to policy analysts, playing on an "uneven playing field." To even stay in the game, they are forced to act like their opponents, which means toughening up their billing and collection practices and managing their indigent patient load. Unfortunately, "managing" is often synonymous with "excluding." An American Hospital Association study found that in 1981 and 1982 about 15 percent of nonprofit hospitals adopted limits on the amount of charity care they provided, and 84 percent increased billing and collection efforts.

There is no question that many tax exempt charitable institutions provided little or no care to the poor well before the proprietary chains came on the scene. For these hospitals, for-profit chains made barring the poor an acceptable way of doing business. For nonprofit hospitals that took their charitable status seriously, the chains made it difficult and in some instances impossible for them to continue fulfilling their mission. The traditional behavior of tax exempt hospitals that provide little or no charity care is being challenged in state courts. A June 1985 decision by the Utah Supreme Court denied tax exempt status to two nonprofit hospitals owned by Intermountain Health Care, a nonprofit hospital chain, because the hospitals did not meet their obligation to provide charity care.

"If you can't beat 'em, join 'em," was a slogan adopted by a large number of voluntary and public hospitals in the early eighties. In addition to conscious efforts to reduce services to the poor, nonprofit hospitals embarked on a mad scramble to buy nursing homes, establish home health agencies, "unbundle" hospital services (remove services such as pharmacy, laboratory, and X-ray from the hospital to get the higher reimbursement rates), specialize in highly profitable ventures such as sports medicine and wellness centers, structure patients care to achieve optimal reimbursement, consider terminating unprofitable services, and advertise.

While most hospitals argue these changes are necessary for survival, others maintain their efforts are directed toward continuing to subsidize charity care. This latter justification is commonly used by public hospitals which began in 1984 and 1985 to undertake corporate restructuring as an alternative to outright sale or transfer of management to a for-profit firm. While the exact configurations vary, the basic idea is to create several new nonprofit and for-profit subsidies. One of the nonprofits will lease the existing hospital for a nominal amount and operate it for the actual public owners, blurring what had once been a clear-cut distinction between for-profit and public hospitals.

Nonprofit hospitals copied the for-profit giants in one other way. Finding strength in numbers, voluntary hospitals began to form their own nonprofit chains. Although some chains of voluntary facilities (such as religious hospitals) predated the rise of for-profit chains, the impetus for increased horizontal integration among nonprofit hospitals in the early 1980s was competition from the proprietary chains.

Good Business or Basic Care?

In 1979, one health analyst commented that "We could wake up in a few years with a few Exxons controlling half the hospitals." It did not take long for this prediction to come true. By 1990, it is likely that ten or so for-profit and nonprofit managed systems will compete with one another to serve the paying customer, while the few public hospitals left (primarily large inner-city facilities which cannot be closed for fear of adverse political repercussions) will continue their struggle to serve the impoverished of the nation. Is this the legacy of the proprietarization of American hospitals? The answer is no. The growth of for-profit chains was simply the natural development of a society that never viewed health care as a right, guaranteed to every citizen, and a government adverse to bucking the prevailing notion that medical providers should be left to their own devices to shape the nation's health care delivery system. If, in the shaping, no space was available for millions of Americans, so be it.

Uwe Reinhardt, a Princeton economist, argues that America's political ideology—its fear of big government—helped to create a medical system that tolerates "visible social pathos in our streets." This system accepts the existence of 35 million uninsured, most of whom are poor and near-poor; denial of prenatal and sometimes delivery care to poor women; the transferring or "dumping" of 500 patients a month from private Chicago hospitals to Cook County General, a public facility; excessive markups on drugs needed to control hypertension and other chronic illnesses; inhuman conditions in many of our nursing homes; and, lately, the premature discharge of elderly patients from hospitals when Medicare payments prove inadequate to cover the costs of care.

Our response to this social pathos depends in large degree on how we view the delivery of medical care. If, as for-profit hospitals maintain, health care is a business, if HCA and Humana are no different than a McDonald's or a Macy's, then our response is obvious: protect against the grossest anticompetitive behavior, but generally adopt a laissez-faire attitude and let market forces dictate the supply and price of goods. If, however, we believe that health care is more than a business, but a societal good, then our response is different indeed. Laws will be needed to assure that prices are controlled, profits limited, and people guaranteed the provision of basic health care.

Which is it? To date, we have either ignored the question or, when forced to confront it, tried to have it both ways. This has led to ambiguous policies at best and huge holes in the nation's health care safety net. The "let's have it both ways" mentality is evident in the government's Medicare policies. Although the provision of medical care to the elderly and disabled is clearly seen as a societal good, the federal government's Medicare reimbursement policy with its substantial return on investment and unlimited passing through of capital costs resulted in huge profits for investor-owned hospital chains and more money going for fewer services. It is only recently, with the advent of DRGs and 1986 legislation to eliminate return on equity (over three years) and proposals to cap federal reimbursements for capital costs, that we have begun to realize that unlimited profits may be at odds with the nation's commitment to providing health care for the elderly.

States have not been any more certain of how to reconcile the needs of the ill and the needs of the medical care marketplace. A few northeastern states have controlled the growth of for-profit hospitals through hospital rate regulation; by limiting rates hospitals can charge, states limit the profits hospitals can make. These states also include payment for care of the indigent in their controlled rates. Other states have sought to require good citizenship of all their hospitals, for-profit and voluntary alike. Florida, South Carolina, and Virginia tax hospitals in order to pay for increased care of the indigent. Tougher emergency room laws in a few states, most notably Texas, have made it more difficult for hospitals to refuse emergency care to the poor or inappropriately transfer them to the nearest public hospital. Efforts have also been made, primarily through the health planning program, to require hospitals wanting to build or modernize to provide a small amount of charity care. North Carolina now requires for-profit hospitals that buy public hospitals to continue to provide care to the poor of the community.

Unfortunately, these efforts are too little too late; the poor and, increasingly, the middle class with inadequate insurance are not guaranteed access to even basic hospital care when ill. Neither the federal government nor the states have been willing to limit profits made from providing hospital care, to require all hospitals to serve a minimum of uninsured and Medicaid recipients, or to provide health care coverage for all in need.

Unlike other Western industrialized nations, we treat medical care as a commodity to be bought and sold in the marketplace.

This marketplace mentality is allowing corporate medicine to distort our medical care system into one that costs us a great deal even while it serves a diminishing share of our people.

PUBLIC PROSPECTS[6]

Public hospitals are as old as the republic, and many of these institutions are facing a crisis in financing that will affect their future. Crisis, particularly financial crisis, is not a new experience for public hospitals, but the current crisis may prove more damaging than many in the past. To cope with the crisis and deal with it effectively, the roots of the current problems must be understood and appropriate policy and management responses initiated.

Approximately one-third of the 5,500 general acute care hospitals in the United State are public hospitals (owned or controlled by a state or local government). These hospitals collectively represent a vital part of our health care delivery system, yet many of them, especially the larger urban public hospitals, are being adversely affected by a number of factors—including the residues of the recession of 1981–82, federal and state health policy changes affecting the organization and financing of health care, and other federal policies (for example, the increased allocation of funds for military purposes) that have limited resources available for domestic social programs. Changes at the state level and in the private sector that have given rise to the wave of enthusiasm for competition in the health care industry are adding to the problems facing public hospitals.

Some public hospitals have closed. Many of the largest remaining public hospitals have reduced their number of beds, cut staffs, postponed capital improvements, and gone back to their local government sponsors for additional financing to maintain their level of service to the poor. In the face of fiscal distress,

[6]Reprint of an article by Robert Hughes, Pew Fellow in health policy at the Institute of Health Policy Studies at the University of California at San Francisco, and Philip Lee, director of the Institute of Health Policy at UCSF. Reprinted by permission from *Society*, 23: 60–65. Jl/Ag '86. Copyright © 1986 by Transaction Publishers.

aging physical facilities, civil service constraints on personnel, and the emerging acceptance of competition and the growth of proprietary enterprises as a rationale for cost containment, public institutions face an uncertain future. The choices available for these hospitals range from closure, sale to proprietary organizations, or creative restructuring, to relying on institutional inertia to see them through the next decade. What is the future role of public hospitals in our health care system?

Hospital ownership falls into three broad types: public, voluntary (private, not-for-profit), and proprietary (private, for-profit). Public hospitals differ from voluntary and proprietary hospitals in important ways. On average, public hospitals are more likely to offer primary medical care services than other hospitals, and they serve people who are poor, less educated, and have less access to physicians than people served by voluntary or proprietary hospitals. These differences are consistent with the historic community role of public hospitals: they are the providers of last resort that care for people who, because of the political and socioeconomic structure of our society, are unable to obtain care elsewhere. Rural public hospitals fill geographic gaps and make services accessible in many sparsely populated areas that would otherwise be acutely underserved. Public hospitals located in cities care for a disproportionately large share of the poor and the uninsured in their communities while other voluntary and proprietary hospitals serve primarily the insured and the nonpoor. Overall, public hospitals fill gaps in our health care system by providing over 17 percent of all hospital care, primarily to the poor and uninsured who would otherwise go without care, be sicker, and die sooner.

Despite their common role as provider of last resort, public hospitals are not homogeneous. The diversity of public hospitals and the roles they played in their communities was an issue addressed by the Commission on Public General Hospitals, established in 1976 by the Hospital Research and Educational Trust (an affiliate of the American Hospital Association). The commission's purpose was "to examine the present health care delivery roles of public general hospitals and to identify future roles, if any, for these hospitals." Recognizing the variation among public hospitals and the need to take account of these differences in assessing their future, the commission divided public hospitals into four groups: (1) urban public general hospitals, or those located in the nation's 100 largest cities; (2) public general hospitals in metropolitan areas outside the 100 largest cities; (3) rural public general hospitals; and (4) university public hospitals.

By far the largest group was the rural public general hospitals, which made up almost three-fourths of all public hospitals. These hospitals, as might be expected, are small (with an average of seventy beds) and provide only 40 percent of the patient days provided in public institutions. They have fewer specialized facilities than other hospitals, fewer physician specialists on staff, and are often the only hospital serving the community in which the hospital is located. The large number of small rural hospitals makes them an important part of our health care system, but they are sufficiently different from large urban public hospitals that it is appropriate to consider their futures separately. These rural public institutions are more likely to be influenced by their monopoly status—that is, by being the sole source of inpatient primary and secondary care in a geographical area with their diverse clientele (not just the poor)—than by the factors that are adversely affecting large, urban public institutions, which, in part, stem from their location in communities with many other hospitals and from their role as major providers of inpatient and outpatient care for the indigent.

The other three groups of hospitals identified by the commission were the large urban public general hospitals (90), the medium-sized metropolitan public general hospitals (357), and the hospitals owned by public universities (45). The commission's report argued that the future of these three groups was likely to be different from each other. The medium-sized metropolitan public hospitals, many of them district hospitals, were found to be similar in many respects to private hospitals in the same settings—in size, financial health, and proportion of paying patients—and thus were not expected to encounter obstacles different from those encountered by such hospitals generally. University owned hospitals were distinguished by the extent to which their future depended on societal decisions about financing graduate medical education and the future role of complex, higher cost tertiary care technology in health care. Their educational and research roles, as well as their specialized tertiary care role, are likely to be the overriding determinants of their future.

The remaining hospitals, the large urban public hospitals, have attracted the most attention from policymakers and others, including the commission. These hospitals are large (with an average of 503 beds) and have traditionally served as provider of last resort in their communities. The report of the commission summarized their situation:

> By tradition, these hospitals serve many patients who have no other source of financing for their health care. They also serve many neighborhood residents for whom they are the hospital of choice, and they frequently provide the community as a whole with certain highly specialized and emergency services. As a group, the urban public-general hospitals are extremely susceptible to financial problems because they serve large numbers of unsponsored patients and provide many services, including ambulatory care services, that are not adequately reimbursed by third-party payers. Many of these hospitals today are in serious financial difficulty because of inadequate local government appropriations and a growing caseload of unsponsored patients. Further, a number of them are encumbered with outdated and outmoded plant and equipment. Because of their weak financial position, they have difficulty in raising capital, even for renovations to bring them into compliance with fire and life safety codes. Many of these urban public hospitals are engaged in training large numbers of physicians and other health professionals, and their medical staffs often are composed of full-time attending physicians who, with medical residents, provide physician services.
>
> Among all hospitals, the urban public-general hospitals, as a group, have the most serious and persistent problems.

Why did these hospitals emerge as a major focus of the commission's work and why do they continue to attract a disproportionate share of policy attention today? In large part it is because their role, which has its roots in their historical mission of providing care to patients regardless of their ability to pay, has resulted in these hospitals absorbing the costs generated by the structural defects of our health care system and of our fragmental system of health care financing. The stresses on these institutions are accentuated by the changes in financing affecting all hospitals.

Urban Crisis

The most fundamental force in the current transformation of our health care system is the effort to control costs. Historically hospitals and physicians have been paid by methods that provided no incentive for efficiency and, indeed, often provided incentives for delivering ever more specialized and expensive services. Increasingly sophisticated technology, potential malpractice suits, rising public expectations, hospital market structure, and the nature of hospital-physician relationships, in combination with perverse economic incentives contributed to health care expenditures absorbing an increased share of the gross national product, particularly during the past twenty years. During this period, the organization of health care was relatively unconstrained by lack of external resources. Physician supply increased rapidly. Physicians continued to practice in relatively the same way and in the same settings as in the past; hospitals, although perhaps inconvenienced by regulatory efforts such as Certificate of Need and health planning programs, for the most part did not significantly alter their organization or financing, and many were able to modernize, expand, and add new services. Financing mechanisms adopted during this period often were designed to accommodate the professional interest groups of physicians and hospitals.

Recently, vigorous efforts to control costs have forced hospitals and (to a lesser extent) physicians to examine their organization and financing with an eye toward responding to externally imposed constraints. These constraints have emanated primarily from government, other third party payers, and employers who have paid for their employees' health insurance. The federal government's implementation of the prospective payment system for Medicare, based on diagnosis related groups, has been important not only for its actual financial consequences, but because it symbolized the extent to which organizations external to hospitals have taken action to explicitly influence hospital behavior. Such actions include selective contracting, utilization review, preadmission screening, prospective pricing, and monitoring lengths of stay; collectively these have been aimed primarily at the costs of inpatient hospital care.

One consequence of these cost-control actions has been a reappraisal of the ways hospitals have allocated the costs of providing care to patients who cannot pay. Approximately 17 to 25 percent of the United States population under sixty-five years of age are uninsured or underinsured, and these people have more need of health care than the general population. In the past they often received care, and the costs were covered internally within hospitals through cost shifting. By increasing charges to paying patients, hospitals can offset the costs of caring for nonpaying patients, as long as they have a relatively large number of paying patients and a small number of nonpaying patients.

In theory, costs for nonpaying patients could be distributed across other citizens through insurance if all participated in the same group insurance, or across the entire population via national health insurance. In fact, these costs have been covered intrainstitutionally via cost shifting, with the hospitals performing the social function of redistributing costs. As third party payers became more active in cost-control efforts, they began to negotiate with hospitals on price and to limit cost shifting, thus forcing hospitals to critically reexamine their traditional ways of financing care for the poor. Hospitals began to pay much more attention to the proportion of their budget devoted to charity care or covering bad debts. Patients who require charity care or who appear likely to incur debts that they cannot repay become a severe institutional liability in such a climate. Increasingly these patients are referred to public hospitals for care.

These organizational and financial changes have adversely affected the large urban public hospitals in two ways. First, the hospitals serve a disproportionate share of nonpaying patients so they are the most affected by restrictions on internal cross-subsidization and the increased "dumping" of nonpaying patients by private hospitals. Second, their historic role as "provider of last resort" has put them at risk of attracting even more nonpaying patients as other hospitals take actions to control their own costs by reducing their numbers of nonpaying patients. These adverse effects are magnified as the federal government seeks to reduce its Medicaid responsibility for financing health care for the poor. Cost shifting has moved from intrainstitutional to interinstitutional, with the costs of providing care to nonpaying patients exported to large urban public hospitals. They are the safety valve for nonpaying patients and other hospitals in their communities, and they are increasingly taking on the burdens generated by the systemic changes in health care financing.

Many public hospitals are financially subsidized to some extent by the government that controls them. A county hospital, for example, might operate at a deficit for the year, with a county board making up the difference through an annual appropriation. Revenue from sources such as Medicaid, Medicare, other third party payers, and patients often falls short of expenses. The changes described have increased such deficits, putting even more pressure on public hospitals to seek additional funds via appropriation, yet at a time when many of their government sponsors are unable to afford increased subsidies. This has caused many governments to seek alternate means of operating their hospitals or, more drastically, to find ways of getting hospitals out of their budgets altogether. Some governments have contracted with private firms to take over management of their hospitals; other public hospitals have been sold outright to private organizations; and still other hospitals have undergone a corporate reorganization that established a new governance mechanism (and budgetary responsibility) independent of the former governmental sponsor.

The current difficulty of the large urban hospitals that have remained public are a result of their role in the overall system of health care, a role that has been advantageous to other hospitals, medical schools, and many third party payers. Systemic costs for indigent care have been exported to these hospitals—the last resort not only for patients, but for other local institutions that, by dint of the existence of a public hospital, are not faced with the unavoidable demands of providing for the poor.

Efforts to control health care costs are inextricably linked to access in our decentralized, pluralistic health care system. As individual hospitals and multihospital systems take steps to ensure their own long-term financial viability, they make strategic decisions that determine the types of patients that will have access to their institutions. For example, a decision to locate a new hospital in an affluent suburban area, to offer services more likely to attract insured patients, or to institute a rigid credit and collection policy—these decisions foster paying patients and discourage nonpaying patients. More subtle, but not necessarily less powerful, forces also affect the payment status of patients likely to use that hospital, such as the extent to which patients who appear indigent are treated with respect and a hospital's reputation for serving anyone in the community.

Actions by individual private hospitals or hospital systems that respond to cost controls in a reasonable way to assure their fiscal viability have the consequence of eroding the fiscal viability of public institutions and reducing access to the system as a whole. The dilemmas facing large urban public hospitals are a consequence of their role relative to other hospitals in the communities and changes in the environment of hospitals generally. Their problems do not stem primarily from internal hospital characteristics such as mismanagement, civil service constraints, demands of unionized workers, or the inefficiencies of bureaucratic medicine; they are overwhelmingly the consequence of factors external to hospital operation—changes in the financial and organizational structure of our health care industry and in the ideas our society has apparently accepted as a rationale for behavior among health care institutions.

The Reagan administration has lead the ideological shift affecting health care through two main themes: New Federalism and competition. New Federalism has emphasized the responsibility of state and local governments for many functions that had increasingly been performed by the federal government over the past forty years. The administration's policies and legislative initiatives have been, in theory, designed to reverse this shift of responsibility. Competition has been adopted as the most appropriate means of distributing goods and services, including health care, within a classic market model. This model encourages discussion of health care primarily in economic terms, using economic concepts such as market share, price competition, and marketing. Health care is viewed increasingly as a commodity purchased from profit-maximizing firms that are part of an industry, and less as a service expected to be available to all citizens. We do not share the Reagan administration's confidence in competition as the most appropriate means to assure access and control costs. The combination of New Federalism and procompetition policies in health care have had the predictable effects of putting strain on the local institutions that provide care for citizens unable to enter into the competitive market because they lack the means: urban public hospitals serving the poor. Medicaid policies, although not the same in all states, often add to the problems facing local public hospitals.

Medicaid is a federal-state assistance program that finances care for low-income blind, aged, disabled, or welfare family members. The Omnibus Budget Reconciliation Act of 1981, legislation whose content was predominantly dictated by the Reagan administration, resulted in federal Medicaid payment reductions of 3 percent in 1982, 4 percent in 1983, and 4.5 percent in 1984. More than one million citizens, primarily the working poor and their children, lost Medicaid eligibility between 1981 and 1985. Of the 20 million people covered by Medicaid, most still have less coverage than citizens with conventional third party insurance; indeed, the extent of that coverage varies markedly from state to state, and it does not begin to address the problem of poor or uninsured citizens whose incomes put them above governmental definitions of poverty or who are excluded through other restrictive criteria. Medicaid now covers only about 40 percent of Americans living in poverty.

Federal policy since 1981 has simultaneously increased the number of citizens without means to pay for care, transferred responsibility for these citizens to state and local governments, and encouraged private sector competition for paying patients. Paying patients are primarily those insured through their place of employment, with the employer paying most of the premium. Urban public hospitals care for a disproportionate share of Medicaid patients, and these patients do not change institutional providers when their benefits are cut or when the state reduces the level of payment to hospitals as it has in California and other states. Medicaid patients that become ineligible may seek care at the public hospital because they know they will receive care regardless of their ability to pay.

Urban public hospitals are facing a crisis generated by reduction in federal programs, limits on local revenues, increased demands for services to people who cannot pay, and the transformation of all facets of health care delivery into an industry dominated by corporate actors. Underlying these changes is an apparent shift in societal values. This is toward acceptance of a federal government overwhelmingly preoccupied with controlling its own spending on health care and away from expectations that governmental policies will be directed at alleviating this country's major inequities in access—inequities unsurpassed in any developed country. Given the current situation, how can large urban public hospitals survive and prosper in the coming decade?

Urban Strategies

Discussions about the fate of large urban public hospitals are not new. Their current situation, fueled by increases in uncompensated care, is even more precarious than in the past. One result of the dramatic increase in the number of uninsured or underinsured patients requiring care, with the increased burden on public hospitals, has been a growing national and state focus on the issue of financing health care for the poor. This has moved to the top of many state and local policy agendas. The survival of the large urban public hospital is tied directly to state and national responses to this issue. Without adequate levels of payment for those who are uninsured or underinsured, large public hospitals cannot survive except as second-rate institutions providing less and less adequate care for the poor.

Health care funding for low-income citizens is essential for these hospitals. The preferable source of this money and the mechanisms of collection and distribution will vary by state and locality, and urban public hospitals will need to adopt approaches tailored to their particular situation. Regardless of the mechanisms, increased funding to pay for these services should be the primary objective of those trying to save these institutions. At both federal and state levels, large urban public hospitals should work collectively and use their firsthand knowledge of the inequities caused by inadequate funding and their access to the political process to press for a resolution. They should rely on the value of equity in our society and demonstrate the inequities that do exist with strategically selected concrete examples. The current crisis of uncompensated care should be used to educate the public about the hospitals' unique community role.

Previous analyses of the problems facing urban public hospitals have concentrated on characteristics of internal management and corporate structure. Such analyses can be considered as a form of institutional victim-blaming. By directing attention to internal difficulties inside the hospitals, these analyses ignore the external factors that are the primary causes of urban public hospital problems. Nevertheless, internal management changes should be considered, but only as part of an overall strategy aimed at increasing the hospital's negotiating power within its local health care system and with state and local government agencies that provide much of their funding. The success that does come from internal management changes and corporate reorganization will depend on how much they help the institution respond to and influence its environment.

Strategies for large urban public hospitals must begin with the recognition that, for many of the institutions, continuing to function in established ways while the environment and other hospitals change will result in additional decline and leave them moribund. Hospital environments are changing drastically. Physician supply is increasing rapidly in many areas of the country. Large employers are forming local and regional health care coalitions to take advantage of their large market shares and control their costs. These coalitions, as well as insurance companies and governments, are negotiating over price and contracting with hospitals and physicians. Health maintenance organizations, preferred provider organizations, and a potpourri of physician-hospital arrangements are proliferating. This realignment and formalization within the health care system will establish its structure for the next several decades. Public hospitals need the ability to operate on an equal basis with their competitors in the organizational, economic, and political processes that will determine their futures.

Within this changing arena, urban public hospitals have the advantage of their traditional mission, which is congruent with deeply held values of equity in our society. But these institutions cannot rely solely on the intrinsic value of their mission. They must also recognize that all health care institutions, even those that clearly provide important services that otherwise would simply not be available, will be subject to economic as well as social criteria of performance.

Governmental agencies and insurers will apply the same economic criteria used to evaluate the performance of private hospitals to public hospitals. The traditional mission of "provider of last resort" will not exempt urban public hospitals from a comparative analysis of performance. They must demonstrate that they have confronted economic issues directly. For example, they should invest effort in strengthening their credit and collections policy by increasing collections from patients who can pay (often via insurance) and developing institutional accounting for those who cannot pay. This will provide the hospital with information about its own operations, which is an essential component of any strategy for change. For example, a large urban public hospital needs a client profile to document its role to politicians, accurate cost data to negotiate with payers, and an accurate description of the amount of charity care and bad debt to get local political credit for the charity care and to demonstrate responsible control of bad debt.

A successful hospital must have management and leadership skills that are directed at influencing governmental policy and negotiating favorable agreements with other organizations. Such leadership and management skills are essential for hospitals to negotiate agreements with physicians, a medical school, other hospitals, insurers, state Medicaid programs, or patient groups. At a national level, this approach has been adopted through the formation of the National Association of Public Hospitals. This organization monitors national legislation that will affect its constituents, testifies at hearings, and works with Congress and its staff to bring the perspective of the large urban public hospitals to bear in the policy process. A similar organization, the California Association of Public Hospitals, has operated on a state level in California.

Despite the bleak current status of large urban public hospitals, they have strengths and characteristics that can be strategically used in establishing their future roles. Many offer services not available at any other hospital. These monopolized services can be the basis of favorable negotiations with other hospitals and payers. The hospitals often have high levels of occupancy (80 to 90 percent) in contrast to declining occupancy in many community hospitals; and it seems unlikely that politicians will close the doors on a hospital that is full of the sick and injured. A hospital full of patients can be an effective bargaining tool in an era of excess hospital-bed capacity.

Bargaining implies an entrepreneurial orientation, and this may seem to contradict the role of these institutions; but an entrepreneurial orientation is not necessarily inconsistent with the traditional values of large urban public hospitals. Such an orientation simply recognizes that effective management and leadership of these institutions will require skills that fit a competitive environment. It does not mean that individual leaders or the hospitals must adopt profit as a primary purpose. Women and men who both possess these skills and are committed to the traditional role of these institutions could, if given the opportunity, have a major impact on the future of these hospitals. Important as such strategic actions by the hospitals themselves may be, the future of public hospitals as a valuable health resource for our country does not rest ultimately on their actions: it rests on the historical resolution of our society's ambivalence toward health care.

Two views of health care have been at the heart of this country's unprecedented expansion and operation of health care delivery during the past several decades, and these views contain opposing answers to the basic questions concerning the government's role in health care delivery. In one view, health care is placed squarely in the context of this country's political economy. The economic characteristics of delivering health care are given primacy, and the dominant criterion by which health care is judged is efficiency. This view of health care underlies most of the cost control efforts initiated in the public sector in the last decade; it also underlies corporate decision making in the vast private proprietary component of health care delivery. In the other view, health care is placed squarely in the moral sphere; it is a right. The obligation of a society toward its members is given primacy in this view, and the dominant criterion for our health care system is equality of access.

Each view emphasizes different aspects of health care, either economic or moral, and each has logical implications when extended into the other's sphere. The economic view, which in this country's ideological heritage means competition, implies that health care should be provided on the basis of ability to pay. Conversely, the logical extension of the view that health care is a right allows for no legitimate principle by which to allocate limited resources. Each view, when logically extended into the opposite sphere, implies a perspective unacceptable to most Americans—that no limits should be put on costs for health care or that health care should be rationed by ability to pay.

Both views are based on values at the heart of American culture: on the one hand, equity; on the other hand competition and merit. Neither view of health care has gained sway over the other, and as a result they both have contributed to, and been strengthened by, an expanding health care market. They grew side by side, opposite in principle, but seldom forced to reconcile. By the late 1970s, the disproportionate expansion of the health care sector within the United States economy generated a demand for fundamental shifts in health care delivery. Reconciling the two views of health care—as a right and as a business—is a need most acutely felt in urban public hospitals. They are the institutional representation of a fundamental value conflict in our societal views of health care, and their future can be watched as a symbol of our country's attempt to resolve the contradictions in economic and moral perspectives of health care.

III. CARING FOR THE ELDERLY

EDITOR'S INTRODUCTION

Although the problem of health care is of concern to everyone, it is especially so for the elderly. The problem of providing for the elderly is made more difficult by the fact that in the last few decades people have been living longer. Breakthroughs in medicine have created cures for diseases that have previously been fatal and have brought other serious illnesses under control. However, the increasing size of the aged population has also resulted in an enormous burden on the health care system, making up a substantial share of its costs. Ethicist in the medical community and the articles in this section discuss how far is too far when caring for the elderly and debate the question of equity in health care cost for those of different age groups.

Every year thousands of elderly citizens and their families wrestle, often unsuccessfully, with the astronomical cost of health care and hospitalization. In 1988, Congress, by an overwhelming majority passed the Medicare Catastrophic Coverage Act intended, it was said, to help alleviate the burden of health care costs. The act provided the elderly with extended coverage for hospitalization, doctors bills and prescription drugs. It's passage set off a fiery debate, with its supporters hailing it as nothing less than a revolution in modern day health care and its detractors denouncing it as a thinly veiled tax increase which unfairly taxed wealthier senior citizens who were already insured for the new services the Act would provide. It was in fact this small group of wealthier senior citizens, who protested bitterly against the bill and precipitated its repeal by Congress in October of 1989. Many of the articles in this section, although written before the Act's repeal, reflect the intense controversy surrounding the issue of who should pay for the health care for the elderly.

In the opening article, Daniel Callahan, writing in *The Nation*, takes the position that a policy of indefinite extension of life through the latest technology, even if it were possible, is economically unfeasible. He argues that seniors who have lived a "natural lifespan," i.e. into their late 70s or early 80s, should not be given life-extending treatment. A following article by Amitai

Etzioni, also in *The Nation,* is a rebuttal to Callahan's proposal. Among the flaws he notes in Callahan's argument is the problem of determining a "natural lifespan," which is viewed differently today than it had been even a few decades ago. Moreover, in a severely depressed economy the definition of elderly could be scaled back to 65 or even younger so as to reduce the health expenditure burden. More than this, the proposal would advantage the rich, who could afford expensive treatment while the average person or the poor could not. Etzioni argues that many other practices could be put in place to contain costs rather than to treat the old so harshly and inhumanely.

Following the debate between Callahan and Etzioni, a staff-written article in *USA Today* reports the release of a new projection of the future number of Americans over 65 by the National Institute on Aging. The projection places their number by the year 2040 at 86,800,000, a full 20,000,000 more than predicted by the Census Bureau. Significantly, those aged 85 or older will constitute almost double the number originally envisioned. How to cope with the medical needs of the increasing number of seniors in our society is the subject of several other articles that follow. In *U.S. News & World Report,* Lisa J. Moor points out a recent trend in elder care is the establishment of day-care centers for the aged who are too frail to stay at home alone but who do not need constant care. A final article in *Ms.* by Grace W. Weinstein discusses the difficulties of the offspring of the elderly who provide care for them at home. Most of these care providers are women, who as yet have had no assistance or financial support to help them in their service to their parents, and are often emotionally and physically exhausted by the experience. As Weinstein notes, proposals for aid to the at-home care providers are being considered both in long-term care insurance and expanded coverage under Medicare.

LIMITING HEALTH CARE FOR THE OLD[1]

In October 1986, Dr. Thomas Starzl of Presbyterian University Hospital in Pittsburgh successfully transplanted a liver into a

[1]Reprint of an article by Daniel Callahan, author and director of the Hastings Center. Daniel Callahan, Limiting Health Care for the Old, *The Nation* magazine/The Nation Company, Inc., copyright 1987. Reprinted by permission.

76-year-old woman, thereby extending to the elderly patient the most technologically sophisticated and expensive kind of medical treatment available (the typical cost of such an operation is more than $200,000). Not long after that, Congress brought organ transplants under Medicare coverage, thus guaranteeing an even greater range of this form of lifesaving care for older age groups.

That is, on its face, the kind of medical progress we usually hail: a triumph of medical technology and a newfound benefit provided by an established health care program. But at the same time those events were taken place, a government campaign for cost containment was under way, with a special focus on health care to the aged under Medicare. It is not hard to understand why. In 1980 people over age 65—11 percent of the population—accounted for 29 percent of the total American health care expenditures of $219.4 billion. By 1986 the elderly accounted for 31 percent of the total expenditures of $450 billion. Annual Medicare costs are projected to rise from $75 billion in 1986 to $114 billion by the year 2000, and that is in current, not inflated dollars.

Is it sensible, in the face of the rapidly increasing burden of health care costs for the elderly, to press forward with new and expensive ways of extending their lives? Is it possible even to hope to control costs while simultaneously supporting innovative research, which generates new ways to spend money? Those are now unavoidable questions. Medicare costs rise at an extraordinary pace, fueled by an increasing number and proportion of the elderly. The fastest-growing age group in the United States is comprised of those over age 85, increasing at a rate of about 10 percent every two years. By the year 2040, it has been projected, the elderly will represent 21 percent of the population and consume 45 percent of all health care expenditures. How can costs of that magnitude be borne?

Anyone who works closely with the elderly recognizes that the present Medicare and Medicaid programs are grossly inadequate in meeting their real and full needs. The system fails most notably in providing decent long-term care and medical care that does not constitute a heavy out-of-pocket drain. Members of minority groups and single or widowed women are particularly disadvantaged. How will it be possible, then, to provide the growing number of elderly with even present levels of care, much less to rid the system of its inadequacies and inequities, and at the same time add expensive new technologies?

The straight answer is that it will be impossible to do all those things and, worse still, it may be harmful even to try. It may be so because of the economic burdens that would impose on younger age groups, and because of the requisite skewing of national social priorities too heavily toward health care. But that suggests to both young and old that the key to a happy old age is good health care, which may not be true.

In the past few years three additional concerns about health care for the aged have surfaced. First, an increasingly large share of health care is going to the elderly rather than to youth. The Federal government, for instance, spends six times as much providing health benefits and other social services to those over 65 as it does to those under 18. And, as the demographer Samuel Preston observed in a provocative address to the Population Association of America in 1984, "Transfers from the working-age population to the elderly are also transfer away from children, since the working ages bear far more responsibility for childrearing than do the elderly."

Preston's address had an immediate impact. The mainline senior-citizen advocacy groups accused Preston of fomenting a war between the generations. But the speech also stimulated Minnesota Senator David Durenberger and others to found Americans for Generational Equity (AGE) to promote debate about the burden on future generations, particularly the Baby Boom cohort, of "our major social insurance programs." Preston's speech and the founding of AGE signaled the outbreak of a struggle over what has come to be called "intergenerational equity," which is now gaining momentum.

The second concern is that the elderly, in dying, consume a disproportionate share of health care costs. "At present," notes Stanford University economist Victor Fuchs, "the United States spends about 1 percent of the gross national product on health care for elderly persons who are in their last year of life. . . . One of the biggest challenges facing policy makers for the rest of this century will be how to strike an appropriate balance between care for the [elderly] dying and health services for the rest of the population."

The third issue is summed up in an observation by Dr. Jerome Avorn of the Harvard Medical School, who wrote in *Daedalus*, "With the exception of the birth-control pill, [most] of the medical-technology interventions developed since the 1950s have their most widespread impact on people who are past their fifties—the further past their fifties, the greater the impact." Many of the techniques in question were not intended for use on the elderly. Kidney dialysis, for example, was developed for those between the ages of 15 and 45. Now some 30 percent of its recipients are over 65.

The validity of those concerns has been vigorously challenged, as has the more general assertion that some form of rationing of health care for the elderly might become necessary. To the charge that old people receive a disproportionate share of resources, the response has been that assistance to them helps every age group: It relieves the young of the burden of care they would otherwise have to bear for elderly parents and, since those young will eventually become old, promises them similar care when they need it. There is no guarantee, moreover, that any cutback in health care for the elderly would result in a transfer of the savings directly to the young. And, some ask, Why should we contemplate restricting care for the elderly when we wastefully spend hundreds of millions on an inflated defense budget?

The assertion that too large a share of funds goes to extending the lives of elderly people who are terminally ill hardly proves that it is an unjust or unreasonable amount. They are, after all, the most in need. As some important studies have shown, it is exceedingly difficult to know that someone is dying; the most expensive patients, it turns out, are those who were expected to live but died. That most new technologies benefit the old more than the young is logical: most of the killer diseases of the young have now been conquered.

There is little incentive for politicians to think about, much less talk about, limits on health care for the aged. As John Rother, director of legislation for the American Association of Retired Persons, has observed, "I think anyone who wasn't a champion of the aged is no longer in Congress." Perhaps also, as Guido Calabresi, dean of the Yale Law School, and his colleague Philip Bobbitt observed in their thoughtful 1978 book *Tragic Choices*, when we are forced to make painful allocation choices, "Evasion, disguise, temporizing . . . [and] averting our eyes enables us to save some lives even when we will not save all."

I believe that we must face this highly troubling issue. Rationing of health care under Medicare is already a fact of life, though rarely labeled as such. The requirement that Medicare recipients pay the first $520 of hospital care costs, the cutoff of reimbursement for care after 60 days and the failure to cover long-term care are nothing other than allocation and cost-saving devices. As sensitive as it is to the senior-citizen vote, the Reagan Administration agreed only grudgingly to support catastrophic health care coverage for the elderly (a benefit that will not help very many of them), and it has already expressed its opposition to the recently passed House version of the bill [the bill was repealed soon after its passage]. It is bound to be far more resistant to long-term health care coverage, as will any administration.

But there are reasons other than the economics to think about health care for the elderly. The coming economic crisis provides a much-needed opportunity to ask some deeper questions. Just what is it that we want medicine to do for us as we age? Other cultures have believed that aging should be accepted, and that it should be in part a time of preparation for death. Our culture seems increasingly to dispute that view, preferring instead, it often seems, to think of aging as hardly more than another disease, to be fought and rejected. Which view is correct?

Let me interject my own opinion. The future goal of medical science should be to improve the quality of old people's lives, not to lengthen them. In its longstanding ambition to forestall death, medicine has reached its last frontier in the care of the aged. Of course children and young adults still die of maladies that are open to potential cure; but the highest proportion of the dying (70 percent) are over 65. If death is ever to be humbled, that is where endless work remains to be done. But however tempting the challenge of that last frontier, medicine should restrain itself. To do otherwise would mean neglecting the needs of other age groups and of the old themselves.

Our culture has worked hard to redefine old age as a time of liberation, not decline, a time of travel, of new ventures in education and self-discovery, of the ever-accessible tennis court or golf course and of delightfully periodic but thankfully brief visits from well-behaved grandchildren. That is, to be sure, an idealized picture, but it arouses hopes that spur medicine to wage an aggressive war against the infirmities of old age. As we have seen, the costs of such a war would be prohibitive. No matter how much is spent the ultimate problem will still remain: people will grow old and die. Worse still, by pretending that old age can be turned into a kind of endless middle age, we rob it of meaning and significance for the elderly.

There is a plausible alternative: a fresh vision of what it means to live a decently long and adequate life, what might be called a "natural life span." Earlier generations accepted the idea that there was a natural life span—the biblical norm of three score and ten captures that notion (even though in fact that was a much longer life span than was typical in ancient times). It is an idea well worth reconsidering and would provide us with a meaningful and realizable goal. Modern medicine and biology have done much, however, to wean us from that kind of thinking. They have insinuated the belief that the average life span is not a natural fact at all, but instead one that is strictly dependent on the state of medical knowledge and skill. And there is much to that belief as a statistical fact: The average life expectancy continues to increase, with no end in sight.

But that is not what I think we ought to mean by a natural life span. We need a notion of a full life that is based on some deeper understanding of human needs and possibilities, not on the state of medical technology or its potential. We should think of a natural life span as the achievement of a life that is sufficiently long to take advantage of those opportunities life typically offers and that we ordinarily regard as its prime benefits—loving and "living," raising a family, engaging in work that is satisfying, reading, thinking, cherishing our friends and families. People differ on what might be a full natural life span; my view is that it can be achieved by the late 70s or early 80s.

A longer life does not guarantee a better life. No matter how long medicine enables people to live, death at any time—at age 90 or 100 or 110—would frustrate some possibility, some as-yet-unrealized goal. The easily preventable death of a young child is an outrage. Death from an incurable disease of someone in the prime of young adulthood is a tragedy. But death at an old age, after a long and full life, is simply sad, a part of life itself.

As it confronts aging, medicine should have as its specific goals the averting of premature death, that is, death prior to the completion of a natural life span, and thereafter, the relief of suffering. It should pursue those goals so that the elderly can finish out their years with as little needless pain as possible—and with as much vitality as can be generated in contributing to the welfare of younger age groups and to the community of which they are a part. Above all, the elderly need to have a sense of the meaning and significance of their stage in life, one that is not dependent on economic productivity or physical vigor.

What would medicine oriented toward the relief of suffering rather than the deliberate extension of life be like? We do not have a clear answer to that question, so longstanding, central and persistent has been medicine's preoccupation with the struggle against death. But the hospice movement is providing us with much guidance. It has learned how to distinguish between the relief of suffering and the lengthening of life. Greater control by elderly persons over their own dying—and particularly an enforceable right to refuse aggressive life-extending treatment—is a minimal goal.

What does this have to do with the rising cost of health care for the elderly? Everything. The indefinite extension of life combined with an insatiable ambition to improve the health of the elderly is a recipe for monomania and bottomless spending. It fails to put health in its proper place as only one among many human goods. It fails to accept aging and death as part of the human condition. It fails to present to younger generations a model of wise stewardship.

How might we devise a plan to limit the costs of health care for the aged under public entitlement programs that is fair, humane and sensitive to their special requirements and dignity? Let me suggest three principles to undergird a quest for limits. First, government has a duty, based on our collective social obligations, to help people live out a natural life span but not to help medically extend life beyond that point. Second, government is obliged to develop under its research subsidies, and to pay for under its entitlement programs, only the kind and degree of life-extending technology necessary for medicine to achieve and serve the aim of a natural life span. Third, beyond the point of a natural life span, government should provide only the means necessary for the relief of suffering, not those for life-extending technology.

A system based on those principles would not immediately bring down the cost of care of the elderly; it would add cost. But it would set in place the beginning of a new understanding of old age, one that would admit to eventual stabilization and limits. The elderly will not be served by a belief that only a lack of resources, better financing mechanisms or political power stands between them and the limitations of their bodies. The good of younger age groups will not be served by inspiring in them a desire to live to an old age that maintains the vitality of youth indefinitely, as if old age were nothing but a sign that medicine has failed in its mission. The future of our society will not be served by allowing expenditures on health care for the elderly to escalate endlessly and uncontrollably, fueled by the false altruistic belief that anything less is to deny the elderly their dignity. Nor will it be aided by the pervasive kind of self-serving argument that urges the young to support such a crusade because they will eventually benefit from it also.

We require instead an understanding of the process of aging and death that looks to our obligation to the young and to the future, that recognizes the necessity of limits and the acceptance of decline and death, and that values the old for their age and not for their continuing youthful vitality. In the name of accepting the elderly and repudiating discrimination against them, we have succeeded mainly in pretending that, with enough will and money, the unpleasant part of old age can be abolished. In the name of medical progress we have carried out a relentless war against death and decline, failing to ask in any probing way if that will give us a better society for all.

SPARE THE OLD, SAVE THE YOUNG[2]

In the coming years, Daniel Callahan's call to ration health care for the elderly, put forth in his book *Setting Limits*, is likely to have a growing appeal. Practically all economic observers expect the United States to go through a difficult time as it attempts to work its way out of its domestic (budgetary) and international (trade) deficits. Practically every serious analyst realizes that such an endeavor will initially entail slower growth, if not an outright cut in our standard of living, in order to release resources to these priorities. When the national economic "pie" grows more slowly, let alone contracts, the fight over how to divide it up intensifies. The elderly make an especially inviting target because they have been taking a growing slice of the resources (at least those dedicated to health care) and are expected to take even more in the future. Old people are widely held to be "nonproductive" and to constitute a growing "burden" on an ever-smaller proportion of society that is young

[2]Reprint of an article by Amitai Etzioni, author and visiting professor at the Harvard Business School. Amitai Etzioni, Health- Care Generation War: Spare the Old, Save the Young, *The Nation* magazine/The Nation Company, Inc., copyright 1988. Reprinted by Permission.

and working. Also, the elderly are viewed as politically well-organized and powerful; hence "their" programs, especially Social Security and Medicare, have largely escaped the Reagan attempts to scale back social expenditures, while those aimed at other groups—especially the young, but even more so future generations—have been generally curtailed. There are now some signs that a backlash may be forming.

If a war between the generations, like that between the races and between the genders, does break out, historians may accord former Governor Richard Lamm of Colorado the dubious honor of having fired the opening shot in his statement that the elderly ill have "got a duty to die and get out of the way." Phillip Longman, in his book *Born to Pay*, sounded an early alarm. However, the historians may well say, it was left to Daniel Callahan, a social philosopher and ethicist, to provide a detailed rationale and blueprint for limiting the care to the elderly, explicitly in order to free resources for the young [see Daniel Callahan, "Limiting Health Care for the Old," *The Nation*, August 15/22, 1987]. Callahan's thesis deserves close examination because he attempts to deal with the numerous objections his approach raises. If his thesis does not hold, the champions of limiting funds available to the old may have a long wait before they will find a new set of arguments on their behalf.

In order to free up economic resources for the young, Callahan offers the older generation a deal: Trade quantity for quality; the elderly should not be given life-*extending* services but better years while alive. Instead of the relentless attempt to push death to an older age, Callahan would stop all development of life-extending technologies and prohibit the use of ones at hand for those who outlive their "natural" life span, say, the age of 75. At the same time, the old would be granted more palliative medicine (e.g., pain killers) and more nursing-home and home-health care, to make their natural years more comfortable.

Callahan's call to break an existing ethical taboo and replace it with another raises the problem known among ethicists and sociologists as the "slippery slope." Once the precept that one should do "all one can" to avert death is given up, and attempts are made to fix a specific age for a full life, why stop there? If, for instance, the American economy experiences hard times in the 1990s, should the "maximum" age be reduced to 72, 65—or lower? And should the care for other so-called unproductive groups be cut off, even if they are even younger? Should countries that are economically worse off than the United States set their limit, say, at 55?

This is not an idle thought, because the idea of limiting the care the elderly receive in itself represents a partial slide down such a slope. Originally, Callahan, the Hastings Center (which he directs) and other think tanks played an important role in redefining the concept of death. Death used to be seen by the public at large as occurring when the lungs stopped functioning and, above all, the heart stopped beating. In numerous old movies and novels, those attending the dying would hold a mirror to their faces to see if it fogged over, or put an ear to their chests to see if the heart had stopped. However, high technology made these criteria obsolete by mechanically ventilating people and keeping their hearts pumping. Hastings et al. led the way to provide a new technological definition of death: brain death. Increasingly this has been accepted, both in the medical community and by the public at large, as the point of demise, the point at which care should stop even if it means turning off life-extending machines, because people who are brain dead do not regain consciousness. At the same time, most doctors and a majority of the public as well continue strongly to oppose terminating care to people who are conscious, even if there is little prospect for recovery, despite considerable debate about certain special cases.

Callahan now suggests turning off life-extending technology for all those above a certain age, even if they could recover their full human capacity if treated. It is instructive to look at the list of technologies he would withhold: mechanical ventilation, artificial resuscitation, antibiotics and artificial nutrition and hydration. Note that while several of these are used to maintain brain-dead bodies, they are also used for individuals who are temporarily incapacitated but able to recover fully; indeed, they are used to save young lives, say, after a car accident. But there is no way to stop the development of such new technologies and the improvement of existing ones without depriving the young of benefit as well. (Antibiotics are on the list because of an imminent "high cost" technological advance—administering them with a pump implanted in the body, which makes their introduction more reliable and better distributes dosages.)

One may say that this is Callahan's particular list; other lists may well be drawn. But any of them would start us down the slope, because the savings that are achieved by turning off the machines that keep brain-dead people alive are minimal compared with those that would result from the measures sought by the people calling for new equity between the generations. And any significant foray into deliberately withholding medical care for those who can recover does raise the question, Once society has embarked on such a slope, where will it stop?

Those opposed to Callahan, Lamm and the other advocates of limiting care to the old, but who also favor extending the frontier of life, must answer the question, Where will the resources come from? One answer is found in the realization that defining people as old at the age of 65 is obsolescent. That age limit was set generations ago, before changes in life styles and medicines much extended not only life but also the number and quality of productive years. One might recognize that many of the "elderly" can contribute to society not merely by providing love, companionship and wisdom to the young but also by continuing to work, in the traditional sense of the term. Indeed, many already work in the underground economy because of the large penalty—a cut in Social Security benefits—exacted from them if they hold a job "on the books."

Allowing elderly people to retain their Social Security benefits while working, typically part-time, would immediately raise significant tax revenues, dramatically change the much-feared dependency-to-dependent ratio, provide a much-needed source of child-care workers and increase contributions to Social Security (under the assumption that anybody who will continue to work will continue to contribute to the program). There is also evidence that people who continue to have meaningful work will live longer and healthier lives, without requiring more health care, because psychic well-being in our society is so deeply associated with meaningful work. Other policy changes, such as deferring retirement, modifying Social Security benefits by a small, gradual stretching out of the age of full-benefit entitlement, plus some other shifts under way, could be used readily to gain more resources. Such changes might be justified prima facie because as we extend life and its quality, the payouts to the old may also be stretched out.

Beyond the question of whether to cut care or stretch out Social Security payouts, policies that seek to promote intergenerational equity must be assessed as to how they deal with another matter of equity: that between the poor and the rich. A policy that would stop Federal support for certain kinds of care, as Callahan and others propose, would halt treatment for the aged, poor, the near-poor and even the less-well-off segment of the middle class (although for the latter at a later point), while the rich would continue to buy all the care they wished to. Callahan's suggestion that a consensus of doctors would stop certain kinds of care for all elderly people is quite impractical; for it to work, most if not all doctors would have to agree to participate. Even if this somehow happened, the rich would buy their services overseas either by going there or by importing the services. There is little enough we can do to significantly enhance economic equality. Do we want to exacerbate the inequalities that already exist by completely eliminating access to major categories of health care services for those who cannot afford to pay for them?

In addition to concern about slipping down the slope of less (and less) care, the *way* the limitations are to be introduced raises a serious question. The advocates of changing the intergenerational allocation of resources favor rationing health care for the elderly but nothing else. This is a major intellectual weakness of their argument. There are other major targets to consider within health care, as well as other areas, which seem, at least by some criteria, much more inviting than terminating care to those above a certain age. Within the medical sector, for example, why not stop all interventions for which there is no hard evidence that they are beneficial? Say, public financing of psychotherapy and coronary bypass operations? Why not take the $2 billion or so from plastic surgery dedicated to face lifts, reducing behinds and the like? Or require that all burials be done by low-cost cremations rather than using high-cost coffins?

Once we extend our reach beyond medical care to health care, if we cannot stop people from blowing $25 billion per year on cigarettes and convince them to use the money to serve the young, shouldn't we at least cut out public subsidies to tobacco growers before we save funds by denying antibiotics to old people? And there is the matter of profits. The high-technology medicine Callahan targets for savings is actually a minor cause of the increase in health care costs for the elderly or for anyone— about 4 percent. A major factor is the very high standard of living American doctors have, compared to those of many other nations. Indeed, many doctors tell interviewers that they love their work and would do it for half their current income as long as the incomes of their fellow practitioners were also cut. Another important area of saving is the exorbitant profits made by the nondoctor owners of dialysis units and nursing homes. If we dare ask how many years of life are enough, should we not also be able to ask how much profit is "enough"? This profit, by the way, is largely set not by the market but by public policy.

Last but not least, as the United States enters a time of economic constraints, should we draw new lines of conflict or should we focus on matters that sustain our societal fabric? During the 1960s numerous groups gained in political consciousness and actively sought to address injustices done to them. The result has been some redress and an increase in the level of societal stress (witness the deeply troubled relationships between the genders). But these conflicts occurred in an affluent society and redressed deeply felt grievances. Are the young like blacks and women, except that they have not yet discovered their oppressors—a group whose consciousness should be raised, so it will rally and gain its due share?

The answer is in the eye of the beholder. There are no objective criteria that can be used here the way they can be used between the races or between the genders. While women and minorities have the same rights to the same jobs at the same pay as white males, the needs of the young and the aged are so different that no simple criteria of equity come to mind. Thus, no one would argue that the teen-agers and those above 75 have the same need for schooling or nursing homes.

At the same time, it is easy to see that those who try to mobilize the young—led by a new Washington research group, Americans for Generational Equity (AGE), formed to fight for the needs of the younger generation—offer many arguments that do not hold. For instance, they often argue that today's young, age 35 or less, will pay for old people's Social Security, but by the time that they come of age they will not be able to collect, because Social Security will be bankrupt. However, this argument is based on extremely farfetched assumptions about the future. In effect, Social Security is now and for the foreseeable future overprovided, and its surplus is used to reduce deficits caused by other expenditures, such as Star Wars, in what is still an integrated budget. And, if Social Security runs into the red again somewhere after the year 2020, relatively small adjustments in premiums and payouts would restore it to financial health.

Above all, it is a dubious sociological achievement to foment conflict between the generations, because, unlike the minorities and the white majority, or men and women, many millions of

Americans are neither young nor old but of intermediate ages. We should not avoid issues just because we face stressing times in an already strained society; but maybe we should declare a moratorium on raising new conflicts until more compelling arguments can be found in their favor, and more evidence that this particular line of divisiveness is called for.

DAY CARE FOR THE ELDERLY[3]

Nearly a third of all working adults now take some responsibility for an older relative—and the number will multiply as the over-80 population mushrooms. In the past, such a commitment has meant putting your loved one in a nursing home, hiring costly home help or giving up your daily routine to do the job yourself. These days, however, adult-day-care centers can often fill the need for a cheaper and less disruptive alternative. More than 1,500 adult-day-care centers—up from a dozen or so in 1970—now serve over 60,000 people.

Care and crafts. Adult-day-care centers serve people too frail to stay home alone but who don't need constant care. Most are open 9 to 5, but some have flexible hours to accommodate work schedules. The two basic kinds of centers are social and medical. Often housed in a YMCA or church, social centers cater to relatively healthy clients with minor impairments. These centers should be run by a nurse or social worker and offer physical and mental stimulation such as exercise, crafts and group discussions. They also should have physical therapists on contract or referral to aid stroke victims. Elderly people with acute health needs—dementia or severe arthritis, for example—probably need a medically oriented center that is generally affiliated with a hospital or nursing home and staffed by a registered nurse, counselors and therapists, with physicians available for consulting. The staff-to-client ratio should not exceed 1 to 8, and staff should monitor client progress and consult with family members. You should expect at least one hot meal a day and transportation to the center and to medical appointments. Many centers can also provide or arrange psychological, podiatric, optometric, dental and dietary care, and

[3]Reprint of an article by Lisa J. Moore, staff writer for *U.S. News & World Report.* Copyright, Sept. 12, 1988, U.S. News & World Report. Reprinted by Permission.

some offer specialized care for those with specific medical needs, such as patients with Alzheimer's disease.

Tallying the costs. The National Council on the Aging puts the average cost of adult day care at $27 to $31 a day, depending on location and services offered. Medical centers may run beyond $80 a day, and transportation may add $7 or so a day. While significant, these expenses are still less than you'd likely pay for a nursing home, which runs at least $79 a day, or for private nursing care, which could cost from $15 to $30 an hour or more. Medicare rarely covers adult day care. Some insurance companies will reimburse a portion of such expenses under long-term health-care plans designed mainly to defray nursing-home costs. Aetna, for example, has an individual plan that pays 50 percent of the nursing-home benefit toward adult day care for up to a year under certain conditions and only following a nursing-home stay. The Travelers offers a plan through employers that pays an amount for adult day care equal to half of the nursing-home benefit, up to $75,000. The monthly cost depends on the age of the relative who one day may need care; it's $68.50 for someone age 65.

Knowing where to look. Though 42 states have standards of quality for adult-day-care centers, fewer than half require licensing. So it's best to visit a center first. You can begin the search by calling your area agency on aging, or by calling the local health or social-services department. Helene MacLean's book, "Caring for Your Parents: A Sourcebook of Opinions and Solutions for Both Generations" (Doubleday & Company), is a thorough guide to adult day care, home care and nursing homes. It's available in bookstores for $12.95 in paperback or $22.50 hard-bound.

THE CONCEPT THAT REVOLUTIONIZED NURSING HOME MARKETING[4]

Mark Twain once said, "A man with a new idea is a quack until he succeeds; then he is considered a genius." Since 1980, George

[4]Reprint of an article by Greg Nielsen, columnist on health care for Vierling Associates International, Inc., a health care marketing and advertising company. Reprinted from USA TODAY MAGAZINE, Nov. copyright 1985 by the Society for the Advancement of Education.

Molloy, president of M&M Associates, the nation's leading health care merchandising firm, has been developing and implementing the dynamic and highly successful "Club Concept" for nursing homes. Now approaching the 500th Club opening, the Club Concept and its creator have not only shaken the industry, they have revolutionized it.

Back in 1980, the nursing home industry had a hard time accepting Molloy's premise. It was wedded to the *status quo;* all patients, private and Medicaid, received the same thing. Nursing home operators did not understand Molloy's attempt to give more to those who paid more simply because they paid more. The operators routinely thought that they should treat everybody equally. At the same time, they treated the private paying patients unequally. Those who paid $5 or $10 more per day did not get $5 or $10 more value for their money. Instead, nursing home operators routinely subsidized the inadequate Medicaid reimbursement by overcharging the private paying patients.

When Molloy stepped into this situation, he was very familiar with the problems of operating and managing nursing homes, having begun administrating a nursing home at the beginning of the Medicare/Medicaid program. In October, 1966, he left a management training program at Dunn & Broadstreet in New York to become the executive director of a new 120-bed extended care facility in Connecticut. In 1969, he moved to New York and became the administrator of a 170-bed skilled nursing home and remained there until 1979, when he began to take a series of management contracts. He managed a 350-bed nursing home in California, a 200-bed facility in Kansas City, and finally a 550-bed nursing home in Pennsylvania.

His knowledge of the day-to-day nursing home operation was the foundation for his merchandising and marketing strategy. For the first time, someone who had an in-depth knowledge of the working details and problems of a nursing home was able to put together a marketing program that would address the provider's, as well as the patient's, problems. Until Molloy, most marketing consultants were from *outside* the nursing home industry.

What is the Club Concept? Basically, it is the practice whereby the nursing home offers the private paying patient a *choice*. The patient or family chooses the Club Plan, then the nursing home gives the Club member 100 additional conveniences, amenities, and services that are not covered by the Medicaid reimbursement. Those patients freely electing to join the Club pay a little more per day, but they receive much more for their money. However, the quality of care remains at the same high level throughout the facility.

For the first time, nursing homes were able to offer the consumer a true choice. Molloy's philosophy was: "Private patients buy . . . they purchase with their own money . . . they select! Medicaid patients *qualify* . . . they qualify for whatever the Federal and state regulations say or dictate they will get."

A momentous legal decision handed down on April 26, 1983, opened the floodgates on the side of private paying patients receiving more than the Medicaid. This justified Molloy's position, which he had advocated since 1980, almost two and a half years before Magistrate Brian P. Short of the United States District Court, Third Division, Minnesota, wrote:

> Nursing homes have maintained throughout these proceedings that they have a right to subsidize the allegedly inadequate Medicaid rate by overcharging the private paying patient . . . this court finds no such right . . . the rate equalization formula promotes a fundamental notion of fairness that one should pay equal rates for equal services. There is no due process right for nursing homes to charge private paying patients a higher rate than the Medicaid rate for the *same services*! [emphasis added]

A Two-Class Hospital System

In recent years, nursing homes have become dangerously dependent on Medicare and Medicaid reimbursement. Nationwide estimates vary, but, for the most part, 70% of the nursing home population is made up of Medicaid patients. The nursing home industry simply did not have a strategy to attract and retain private pay. Although it needed private paying patients, it could not and did not attract them because, as Molloy said, "there was no incentive for an affluent private paying patient to enter a nursing home, pay more, and receive what the Medicaid or welfare patients were getting!"

A recent article in *Business Week* quoted political economist E. Reinhardt of Princeton University:

> I think we will end up with a two-class hospital system. For the affluent and well-to-do, we will have luxurious hospitals with great amenities. For the publicly financed (Medicare/Medic-

aid), we will have something more like wards—four people in a room with few amenities. That may sound sad, but I think America is firmly moving in that direction.

Reinhardt's comments echoed the views Molloy first stated in 1980.

Molloy was a visionary who had the courage to teach his strategy to long-term care facilities. He pointed out that "The wards of the forties and fifties were replaced by the Medicare and Medicaid credit card of the sixties and seventies. During the same time frame, the private paying, affluent patients, whether in hospitals or nursing homes, always had the means to provide for themselves whatever accommodations and amenities they needed or desired." Medicare and Medicaid could not and did not change that reality.

Now, in the 1980's, Federal and state government officials are finding it more difficult to provide quality health care under the Medicare and Medicaid formula to the degree they had wished and hoped for. Cutbacks and reductions are inevitable. Consequently, in the 1990's, there will be a two-class system of health care. The hospitals know it; the nursing homes are finally understanding it.

Paul Vierling, president of Vierling Associates International, a leading Reno, Nev.-based health care advertising firm, said of Molloy, "I went to one of his strategy workshops. I could not believe the depth of his knowledge about health care, merchandising, and marketing. He was especially brilliant in describing the problems of long-term care facilities. His inside knowledge of how the industry operated proved to be the most essential ingredient for his success in teaching nursing homes a true marketing strategy!"

Since 1980, Molloy has blazed new pathways and directions for the nursing home industry. His strategy is more than a one-time seminar; it is backed up with the most extensive legal research in the country on Federal and state Medicaid regulations. His clients are given an overview of Federal Medicare and Medicaid law and then, in each state, a breakdown of how his Club Concept is valid.

Prior to Molloy, most marketing consultants were teaching a traditional single seminar or workshop. Molloy gave facilities that were his clients a comprehensive over-all strategy. He protected his clients with a one-year written agreement not to teach any competition the workings of his program. He says,

Most market strategies of the past were based on imaging a nursing home—trying to show nursing homes in a more positive light. Such things as rock and roll jamborees [or] Nursing Home Week [were] trying to convince the community that nursing homes were not all that bad, etc. My program focuses on teaching nursing homes how to properly identify their product and then to point out how it is unique, special and different.

His campaign was well-received because of the total strategy involved. First, he works with the staff and sees to it that they fully understand the concept and the reason for it. In addition, he spends a great deal of time with the owners and operators of the facility in providing them with the pricing formula and the amenity lists. Secondly, he works with the admission coordinators to get them to understand some basic sales and interviewing techniques.

Financial information is the most important part of the admission process. Most admissions people are good at getting medical information, but terrible in getting financial information. No other business sells to a customer without a credit or bank check. A department store will not sell a dozen pair of socks on a credit card unless the credit application had financial information to begin with. Nursing homes routinely admit people into $70-a-day rooms and let them run up a bill without any credit check, bank references, or financial data.

One nursing home in a western state had been hard hit by Medicaid cuts in 1982 and 1983. It needed a strategy to attract and retain more private paying patients, since it could no longer make it under the inadequate Medicaid rate. It needed to enhance revenues and to do it quickly. The administrator read about the Club Concept program in a trade journal, contacted Molloy, and requested references. She contacted all the references personally and was impressed with the uniformly positive reports she heard, then attended one of Molloy's public seminars. After hearing the concept explained in detail, she convinced the owner to have Molloy present his in-house program.

Four months after Molloy left, her facility attracted an astounding 100% increase in private paying patients. A well-planned print and radio advertising campaign contributed to the rapid advertising campaign contributed to the rapid acceptance of the Club Concept. The administrator summed up her experience with Molloy's strategy by saying, "There is simply nothing like it. Imagine 100% increase in private paying patients in just a couple of months."

A California facility experienced a staggering 400% increase in private paying patients in six months. The Club Concept was so well-received in that particular community that a government agency referred prospective patients and families to tour the home to see it for themselves. Medicaid patients benefited directly from the increased private paying population. The administrator remarked that the increased revenues meant that they could actually afford to give *more* to the Medicaid patients than previously. "Everybody benefited from the Club," she said. "The staff has seen a very positive improvement. They are supportive and behind the Club 100%. It is absolutely remarkable how comprehensive Molloy's strategy really is. The only way to understand it is to experience it."

Another facility had been devastated by drastic cuts in Medicaid reimbursement and a sudden drop in the Medicaid population. For the first time in eight years of business, they showed a loss. Vacancies were up, and they did not have a plan to counteract a string of unfavorable occurrences. Enter Molloy, who spent two full days with the administrative staff.

The facility had applied for a $500,000 loan in order to expand the number of beds and to help build an adjoining small retirement complex. Molloy met with the bank loan officer and explained that his Club Concept would bring an end to the facility's dependence on an uncertain and unfavorable government handout. It would tap the affluent of the community and make the facility financially independent. After meeting with Molloy, the banker responded, "I am very impressed. The facility will get its money. The Club Concept is a unique and novel idea. I have other retirement homes and nursing homes in trouble. I would like to share this concept with them."

The owners of the facility were elated, not only with Molloy's efforts with the staff of the facility, but also with the bankers. The owner summed up their experience with Molloy by saying, "We were lost before Molloy gave us his strategy. Now we have new hope and vitality."

In another case, an East Coast nursing home opened a Club section on Dec. 1, 1984. By Jan. 10, 1985, 60 private paying patients joined the Club—30 in-house and 30 from outside. Remarkably, one Medicare patient refused benefits in order to join the Club and enjoy the extra conveniences and services. Other government-supplied patients in the same facility are clamoring to join a Club with amenities.

As more Medicare/Medicaid patients refuse benefits to join the Club, state Medicaid budgets will go further for those who are truly needy. As it stands now, there is no incentive for borderline Medicaid patients to elect private pay since, in most nursing homes, Medicaid and private pay patients receive the same. Why pay more for the same? Club offers a clear choice—you pay more, you get more!

The Club Concept actually preceded the Reagan Administration's efforts at trying to instill more competition into health care in general. In a 1984 interview in *Business Week,* Secretary of Health and Human Services Margaret Heckler commented: "The objective in this administration is to produce a more competitive health care marketplace rather than trying to impose on it more regulation. Competition can reduce costs while preserving quality. I personally prefer the free market approach to the bureaucratic straightjacket which total regulation would provide the health care industry."

This sentiment was four years behind Molloy's creative and innovative approach to the nursing home industry. The Club Concept teaches nursing homes how to become more competitive. As he explains,

> If you look at the yellow pages in any city and look at the thousands of dollars spent on yellow pages advertising, you will get sick to your stomach. Consider what those thousands of dollars are doing for a nursing home. They are actually doing nothing except proving my point. Nursing homes are all selling the same things. They all offer something called "skilled" or "intermediate" care—whatever that is. They all have private and semi-private rooms! They all have barber and beautician. They all have a registered dietician.

The secret of merchandising a service is certainly not to have sameness, the fundamental error in nursing home marketing. Molloy's strategy is to teach nursing homes how, with their Club, to be unique, special, and different. A nursing home with a Club is able to give free what other nursing homes charge extra for. The one Club rate includes 100 valuable amenities. Other nursing homes charge extra for what a Club gives for its Club rate. With a Club section of the nursing home, the consumer knows pretty much what the cost will be. There are no monthly surprises whereby the bill goes up and down like a roller coaster. The consumer has a true choice. This is the way to drive out Medicaid mediocrities.

Discrimination and Segregation

The two problems that Molloy routinely faces are the charges of discrimination and segregation. Most of the charges come from Medicaid bureaucrats who know his strategy allows nursing homes to break out of the Medicaid handcuffs of dole and dependence. Molloy is straightforward when he describes discrimination allegations:

Discrimination means showing a prejudice against a person or a class. Why are Medicaid officials so choosy in determining which class of patients they will protect against "discriminatory" practices? Surely, Medicaid officials know that the private paying patients are being forced to pay *twice* for Medicaid. First, by their taxes, and secondly because private paying patients are the victims of cost shifting.

Medicaid officials are not ignorant of the Minnesota rate equalization law. Medicaid officials know that private paying patients have always been discriminated against; yet, these same officials are silent about *that discrimination!*

Molloy is equally blunt discussing segregation:

Segregation means the act of separating from the main body. It is the Medicaid bureaucrats that taught the nursing home industry how to "*segregate*" patients. When the officials do it, it's called certification! The politicians and the bureaucrats conveniently play with words to suit *their purpose*. The segregation of today is nothing more than the certification of yesterday.

At one time, only *certain patients* (skilled or Medicare patients) could be housed and cared for in a certain section of the facility (the certified section). If the nursing home put a Medicare or Medicaid patient in a non-certified section, there would be no reimbursement.

When private paying patients are given a separate or special section, and given accommodations and amenities that they, the private paying patients, pay for, then it is somehow "segregation." If the state does not require total certification of beds, then it is perfectly appropriate to have a distinct part for Club patients. The Medicaid bureaucrats may not like it, but the law allows it.

Some states have only partial Medicaid certification. They use it as a method to hold down Medicaid costs. If a bed is not certified, then, of course, a state doesn't have to pay for it. Talk about discrimination!

One state had its commissioner ranting and raving about the nursing homes setting up "Medicaid ghettos!" These inflammatory remarks were not only totally inappropriate, but when the state Medicaid reimbursement formula was analyzed, everyone could see that the only ones who are creating a "Medicaid ghetto" are the Medicaid reimbursement bureaucrats.

Molloy's concept is forming the basis for nursing homes to be able to break away from Medicaid dependency. More and more state officials acknowledge privately that his focus on the private pay market can actually help them hold down Medicaid costs. For the first time, private paying families and patients have an *incentive* to remain off Medicaid.

In one Club nursing home after another, families and patients appreciate the accommodations, enjoy the amenities, and like to receive more value for their dollar. Under the old system, there was no incentive for patient or family to pay privately. "Why should they," Molloy asks, "when all that they got for their money was the same as the welfare patient? Now under my concept, patients and families are willing to pay for the Club and amenities [and] thus stay off Medicaid. More and more state officials are talking to me about this potential."

Today, the private pay population is the fastest growing segment of the $28,000,000,000-a-year nursing home industry. It is that segment that Molloy targeted in 1980. His advice to the nursing home industry is simple:

Make the Club sections nice, make the Club amenities valuable. Cater to those who purchase with their own money instead of qualifying for the government handout and you will always have a market that will surprise you. It is time for the nursing homes to decide which market they will service. There is room, of course, for both segments. That is exactly why my program has been so successful. I point out to the nursing home industry that, instead of one market, there is really two; and I have given them the strategy and the technique to capture the private pay market.

Prominent in Molloy's office is a plaque that describes his merchandising/marketing philosophy. It sums up the man, the vision, and the concept.

In order to be successful in the nursing home business—we must sell care, treatment, and service at a profit and, at the same time, satisfy our residents. If we satisfy the patients, but fail to get the profit, then we will soon be out of business. If we get the profit, but fail to satisfy the residents, then we will soon be out of patients. Without patients, we will surely be out of business.

The secret of success in the nursing home business is found in *Merchandising!* Merchandising means that they have a *Product* that they are proud of; a product so valuable and appealing for their residents and patients that the residents pay a *Price* which allows the nursing homes to make a *Profit.* By making a profit, the quality nursing homes will remain in business and survive the Medicaid mediocrities.

HELP WANTED—THE CRISIS OF
ELDER CARE[5]

The statistics are staggering:

• One in eight Americans is over age 65. By the year 2030, one in five will be over 65.

• The fastest growing segment of the elderly population consists of men and women (mostly women) over age 85. Fully half of this group requires assistance with daily living due to chronic illness or disability.

• At least 80 percent of the people needing long-term care receive it from family and friends. Social services targeted to this need are few and far between, and help in paying for those services is virtually nonexistent.

• The average woman will spend 17 years caring for children and 18 years caring for aged parents. In between, or simultaneously, she may spend years caring for an ill or disabled spouse.

[5]Reprint of an article by Grace W. Weinstein, contributing editor of *Ms.* magazine. Reprinted with permission from *Ms.*, 18:73–74, 76, 78–79. O '89. Ms. Magazine Copyright 1989.

Sheila Gallagher (not her real name) began to learn the harsh reality behind these statistics when she was awakened one Sunday morning at six by a frantic telephone call from her 77-year-old mother. "She said she'd been waiting for me for dinner for hours, but that was only the beginning," says Gallagher. "Later that day she called into another room to ask my father, who'd been dead for eleven years, whether he was planning to mow the lawn."

You've heard about the "mommy track." Now brace yourself for the "daughter track," identified in a recent study by *Fortune* magazine and John Hancock Financial Services as a path populated by women who devote so much time to care of the elderly, usually a parent, that their careers are threatened. Men care for parents too. But study after study shows that men more often help with the checkbook or keep in touch by telephone. Women provide personal hands-on care: they cook, do housework, administer medicine, shepherd parents to the doctor. They also bathe them, dress them, change them, and feed them. Not infrequently, women provide such care for more than one aging relative—parents, in-laws (sometimes even after divorcing their son), aunts, and, eventually, their own husbands.

"The empty nest is nothing more than a myth," says Lou Glasse, president of the Older Women's League (OWL), referring to the assumption that women who have finished raising children can finally put their own needs first. "If women's nests' empty at all, they fill again very quickly with elderly parents or other relatives who need care and support."

Right now, according to a study sponsored by the American Association of Retired Persons and the Travelers Companies Foundation, up to 7 million people, 75 percent of them women, are providing care for an average of 12 hours a week and have been doing so for at least two years. More than half of these caregivers hold paying jobs, but other studies show that many caregivers, burdened with overwhelming responsibility, give up their jobs or cut back on working hours to the point where they lose out on their own health and retirement benefits. Such "volunteer" caregiving, says Glasse, is "a prime cause of the poverty that so many women endure in old age."

As the saying goes, though, we ain't seen nothin' yet. "Child care is still overshadowing elder care as an issue, and probably will for the next five to seven years," says Dana Friedman of the Families and Work Institute. Like a snake swallowing a mouse, the focus will begin to shift as the parents of the baby boom generation move into their seventies. The oldest baby boomer is now 43, her mother 65. The real crunch, the point at which the need for support services will become obvious to the most myopic politician, will come when the baby boom generation itself is elderly.

The caregiver today, however, has no time to take in the big picture. When Sheila Gallagher's mother began to show signs of dementia—a mental condition compounded, as it often is, by physical problems—she couldn't be left alone. "Mom needed someone to stay with her at night after she became very agitated and wandered two miles away," says Gallagher. "Eventually she needed someone all day." Gallagher tried to function at work while arranging care for her mother. That meant endless hours on the telephone with doctors, day care facilities, and home health agencies—calls that for an employed woman are made at lunchtime. "I've been so stressed out," she said one April day. "I haven't had a day off since November or gone out for lunch more than three times in the last year. It's like another full-time job. It's put a complete stop to my life."

Like many caregivers, Gallagher is doing everything possible to keep her mother at home instead of in a nursing home. Only 5 percent of those over 65 are in nursing homes at any one time because both the elderly and most of their relatives prefer home to institutional care. But marshaling support for home care takes its toll.

Caregivers describe depleted wallets. They also report aching backs and pulled muscles from lifting. Most of all, whether providing hands-on care themselves or supervising paid help, they display emotional fatigue. With less time to spend with their own families, interruptions on the job, postponed vacations, and altered retirement plans, it's little wonder that caregivers suffer from depression, anxiety, frustration, helplessness, sleeplessness, and sheer emotional exhaustion.

They also feel guilt about not doing "enough," and guilt is a great inhibitor. It keeps you from demanding help and makes you personalize the problem. As Stephen McConnell, national coordinator of the Long Term Care Campaign, puts it, "In the past, long-term care was an issue families struggled with quietly in their own homes, out of a sense of guilt and responsibility. They haven't viewed it as something to talk to legislators about." But the need for long-term care services is coming out of the closet and emerging as a hot political issue. It's time to demand help.

Navigating the Maze

The key elements of elder care are nursing homes, home health care, adult day care, and respite services. "Unfortunately," as OWL's Lou Glasse sums up the situation, "very little outside help is available. That which does exist is expensive, of poor quality, or both." Existing services are so inadequate, at least in part, because people can't pay for them; most observers agree that when financing mechanisms are in place, services will follow.

The average annual cost of a nursing home is now $25,000 a year; some cost upward of $50,000 a year. At the same time, the median family income of the elderly is about $20,000 a year, while older women living alone have a median income of about $7,000. Beds are often in short supply, with national occupancy rates exceeding 90 percent. As for quality, although legislation passed by Congress in 1987 set standards of care for nursing homes receiving payment under either Medicare or Medicaid, implementation is lagging. Many provisions won't take effect until October 1990.

Confronting poor care is very difficult, because an elderly resident is vulnerable. "I complained about a nurse, but not as loudly as I might have," says one daughter, "because they have ways to get even. Dinner might be late, or cold, or she might handle my mother a bit more roughly than necessary."

Although 42 states fund limited home care services, OWL reports that the programs serve only about 100,000 Americans while fully one million seriously disabled elderly living at home receive no assistance at all. Many caregivers are forced to place elderly relatives in nursing homes because there is so little support for at-home care.

Even when at-home care is available and affordable, frequent turnover among poorly paid aides often means inadequate care. Home care workers earn so little and receive so few benefits that OWL has adopted their cause. The quality of care is affected as well by the lack of training and, given the isolated work sites, inadequate supervision that aides receive. Here, too, implementation of federal quality-of-care standards is slow. Neither home health aide training provisions nor toll-free home care hotlines are yet in place.

There are long waiting lists for adult day care programs, which can cost up to $50 a day or even more. Only 1,400 such centers exist nationwide, serving 66,000 persons. Many more of the elderly could benefit from the stimulation and socialization found in good day care; many more of their caregivers could benefit from time off.

Time off, in fact, is essential. Respite programs can make it possible for a full-time caregiver to get a haircut, visit the dentist, attend a wedding, take a vacation, retain her sanity. Programs specifically designed as respite for caregivers—as opposed to adult day care, which is designed primarily to benefit the elderly person—can run from an afternoon's at-home visit by a home health aide to a week-long stay in a nursing home. Yet Elaine M. Brody of the Philadelphia Geriatric Center, a *Ms.* Woman of the Year in 1985 known for her research on caregiving and "women in the middle," notes that instead of regular funding for respite programs, there are only "episodic and discontinuous efforts" to provide this sorely needed help.

One of the biggest problems family caregivers face is finding out where to find help. A hospital discharge planner can provide referrals if help is needed immediately after hospitalization. But elderly people often deteriorate without being hospitalized. The endless hours that the Sheila Gallaghers of this world spend on the telephone seeking help can be cut short by what social workers call a single "point of entry" into the system, a person or agency to determine just what services are needed and provide information on where to find them.

The need is spurring the growth of a new profession: private geriatric care managers who assess need, coordinate services, and monitor care. Private care managers, often coming from social work or nursing backgrounds, are particularly helpful when long-distance caregiving is necessary—a service that Rona Bartelstone, a Miami-based care manager, says is typical of her practice." But even when the family is nearby," says Bartelstone, president of the National Association of Private Geriatric Care Managers, "it might need help in knowing the options and establishing the best care plan."

Andi Klein (not her real name), herself a gerontological nurse, turned to a care management company after almost two years of struggling on her own to meet the needs of a widowed father 650 miles away. "I needed someone to find and manage the caregivers," she says. "They did an excellent job of assessing the situation and came up with good candidates for us to interview."

Private care management, which is generally not covered by either Medicare or private insurance, can cost from $60 to $125 an hour, and costs can mount if long-term monitoring of care is needed. But even where money is tight, several hundred dollars for an initial evaluation plus recommendations might be money well spent.

Before you turn to a private care manager, however, you might check with a state or local agency on aging to see what public services exist. In Connecticut, for example, a call to Connecticut Community Care Inc., a private nonprofit agency, can provide one-stop shopping. The agency helped one woman, frantic because her mother was in a nursing home in Florida, transfer her mother to one nearby in Connecticut. An initial evaluation costs $320; time spent in coordinating services and monitoring care is $75 an hour. Because state and federal money provides some of the agency's funding, however, you can place a call for help without first balancing your checkbook. Users may pay privately for services, pay on a sliding scale, or pay through public funds.

Paying for Help—Whose Pocket?

The bottom line, as always, is money. In 1987, according to the Pepper Commission on comprehensive health care, $56 billion was spent on long-term care, a figure that can only grow as cost containment forces patients out of hospitals "quicker and sicker." In 1985, 44 percent of the total spent came from patients and their families, 41 percent from Medicaid, 7 percent from Medicare, with other public funds and insurance picking up the balance.

One of the biggest shocks, as Sheila Gallagher can testify, is finding that Medicare does not cover much of the care the elderly need. By statute, it does not cover custodial care—the day-in, day-out help with ordinary living, whether at home or in a nursing home, that is the essence of long-term care. "I kept increasing the hours of help until it was costing $700 a week," says Gallagher. "It's frightening to see how fast money can go. My poor mother thought she had a little cushion, and it was gone in six months. We had to sell her house to pay for her care."

The Medicare picture may now be just a little brighter. Under the Catastrophic Coverage Act of 1988 [since repealed], 150 days a year (up from 100 days per illness) will be covered in a skilled nursing facility and prior hospitalization will no longer be required. Respite care will also be covered—a scant 80 hours a year but, for the first time, a recognition of the need.

Perhaps more important, according to Robert M. Freedman, a New York attorney who is one of the founders of the National Academy of Elder Law Attorneys, recent court cases have led to a more liberal definition of skilled care, the kind Medicare will pay for. Where Alzheimer's was almost always considered a chronic condition and therefore not eligible for Medicare coverage, for instance, now severely afflicted Alzheimer's patients who require monitoring for medication—perhaps 25 to 30 percent of nursing home patients—could be covered. As a result, Freedman asserts, an appeal of Medicare's denial of benefits may be well worth pursuing.

There are two other financing options, other than your own pocket: private long-term care insurance and Medicaid, the federal/state program for the poor. Long-term care insurance, while much in the news lately, is still not the answer for most people. Too many existing policies require hospitalization prior to nursing home admittance. Newer policies are less restrictive and do cover home health care but are still expensive. The average annual premium for a 65-year-old was $920 in 1988, the Health Insurance Association of America reports; for a 79-year-old it was $3,010.

Farsighted employers, both corporations and state governments, are beginning to provide long-term care insurance for their employees; the employees pay the cost, but the premiums tend to be about 30 percent lower than on individually purchased policies. Some employers also sponsor elder care referral services, and others have counseling programs or leave benefits that are adaptable to long-term care needs. More employers are likely to become involved in elder care (unlike child care) because, as the recent *Fortune*/John Hancock study noted, half of the top executives surveyed have some personal experience with caring for an elderly relative.

Medicaid is another, usually involuntary, financing option. The poor use Medicaid from the start; the middle class turn to Medicaid after "spending down" to poverty levels. It doesn't take long. According to a study by the House Select Committee on Aging, seven out of ten elderly persons living alone found themselves at the poverty level after only 13 weeks in a nursing home. Half of all married couples became impoverished in six months.

Medicaid rules are so stringent that they have been called "victim-based financing." They have led to what OWL terms "spousal impoverishment," the literal hand-to-mouth existence of the well spouse in order to make the nursing home resident eligible for Medicaid. In Florida, a minister made the news recently when he obtained a divorce because it was the only way he could afford to care for his wife. Here, too, there may be some slight improvement for low-income elderly, depending on state legislation, as income and asset ceilings were raised in the Catastrophic Coverage Act.

One problem with financing long-term care is that it's not yet factored into our personal planning; we plan to buy a house, put our children through college, retire someday, but we don't plan on needing long-term care.

Public Policy

If long-term care is provided in the form of a social insurance program like Medicare, the tab is likely to be at least $20 billion a year. Some estimates run to $60 billion. Who's going to pick up the tab? The Catastrophic Coverage Act set a precedent for financing by beneficiaries; it also kicked up a fire storm of protest by older citizens who consider the financing unfair. Proponents of long-term care coverage are faced with the daunting task of devising a way to pay for it that won't generate a similar storm.

But there's a subliminal subtext to the financing issue, centering around how policymakers regard both women and the elderly. Is the country really prepared to replace the unpaid labor of daughters, daughters-in-law, and wives with a paid system of services? Women themselves don't readily relinquish the responsibility. "All the leftover psychological issues surface when a parent is in need," says one daughter, "the whole feeling of should I be doing more." Those feelings can be compounded by cultural taboos; one parent's Cuban heritage, for example, precluded care by anyone but family. Personal feelings aside, as a nation we haven't even managed to pass the Family and Medical Leave Act, which would grant ten weeks of unpaid leave to care for an ill or disabled child or parent; note that spouses aren't included.

Most Americans agree with organizations like OWL that we need support services for caregivers, including widely available respite care, that we need to prevent the impoverishment of the caregiving spouse, and that we need to find some way, as a nation, of paying for long-term care for a rapidly aging population. When asked during the last presidential election whether or not it was "time to consider some kind of government action or insurance program" to support long-term care, registered voters favored government action by nearly 10 to 1.

Policymakers are beginning to sit up and take notice, and several bills have been introduced. As Stephen McConnell of the Long Term Care Campaign describes the measures, they range from the very narrow (incentives to purchase private insurance) through a middle range (the late Congressman Claude Pepper's proposal to extend Medicare coverage to home care) to comprehensive measures (plans to cover both home care and nursing home care through Medicare). The comprehensive bills differ dramatically when it comes to nursing home coverage: Senator Edward Kennedy's bill, for example, would pay in full for the first six months of care, with partial coverage thereafter, while Senator George Mitchell's proposal would provide no coverage at all for the first two years but 70 percent coverage for the long haul. Since relatively few people remain in a nursing home for more than two years, Kennedy's measure would cover more people while Mitchell's would help people who need help the most.

Although these bills and others are in the legislative hopper, no real action is expected until the Pepper Commission, established to investigate both long-term care and access to health care in general, completes its study. A report is expected next March.

This is a good time, therefore, to write to your legislators. Tell them it's time, past time, for women's work as caregivers to be recognized and supported. You might remind them of the folk tale about a mother asking her son to carve a wooden bowl for his elderly grandfather's meals, after the old man's shaking hands had broken many dishes. The son carved two wooden bowls, telling his mother when she asked why, "It's for you, when you get old." We'll all, given luck, grow old. We, then, as our elderly relatives now, deserve to end our days in dignity.

IV. THE NATIONAL HEALTH INSURANCE ISSUE

EDITOR'S INTRODUCTION

One aspect of health care receiving increasing attention is the issue of whether the country should adopt some form of national health insurance. In the past a national health insurance system has been adamantly and widely opposed by many members, groups, and institutions of society, among them the American Medical Association, the insurance industry, and the large corporations. Now, however, with the soaring cost of medical care, the idea of a comprehensive health insurance plan is being reassessed. The opening article in this section, an editorial in *The Progressive,* considers a number of national health insurance proposals, including one advanced by Senator Edward Kennedy, a Federal version of the "Massachusetts plan," which would mandate a minimum level of employer-funded coverage. Another proposal, one favored by conservatives, is a voucher system that would enable all citizens to buy health insurance suited to their needs and circumstances through private insurers. However, both plans, the editorial maintains, would preserve the present "fee-for-service" arrangement and thus would do nothing to contain costs. The voucher system, moreover, would serve the affluent better than the poor, and would transfer more of the burden of health insurance coverage from employers to employees.

The second article, by Carol J. Loomis in *Fortune,* focuses on the mounting burden to corporations of providing health insurance to its workers and retirees. Of particular concern is the cost of retiree benefits which are provided by about 70 percent of all large companies, but which are being severely cut back. Corporations are also deeply troubled by new regulations by the Financial Accounting Standards Board that may go into effect in 1992. These regulations would require companies to charge their health insurance obligations, present and future, to their earnings, which would reduce returns to their shareholders. A related article by Steven Waldman writing in *Newsweek* reports that a National Leadership Commission, made up of business, medical, and political leaders, has endorsed a major restructuring of the nation's health care system that would include a guarantee of basic medical coverage for everyone. The AFL-CIO is also gearing up to launch a major campaign to promote its own plan that would provide universal access to medical care.

The concluding article examines the privately run but government-funded Canadian health insurance system as a possible model for a restructured system in the United States. In an address before the American Medical Association, William E. Goodman, a Canadian physician, discusses the Canadian system in detail and finds it seriously lacking. Canadian expenditures on health care are less than in the U. S., but this is partly because Canadian investment is curtailed in medical technology. In addition, regulations of various kinds reduce availability of treatment. Even those in urgent need of surgery, such as a cardiac bypass, may be placed on a waiting list of months, and may not expedite things by paying for the operation privately. The system is bureaucratic to a degree that Goodman believes would be unacceptable to Americans with their individualistic spirit.

A HEALTHY DEMOCRACY[1]

After more than forty years of stalling, malingering, ducking, and dodging, the American Establishment will finally have to confront the question of national health insurance. The crisis in health care is not just a cliché but an increasingly disruptive factor in the nation's political and economic life. Even that quintessential model of corporate greed, Lee Iacocca, has taken to advocating some sort of Government intervention.

Health insurance costs are an increasingly abrasive issue in labor negotiations in both the private and public sectors as more workers are being asked to pick up some or all of the premiums. The number of workers having no coverage at all is rising. Among the poor, those covered by Medicaid have declined from a high of 63 per cent in the mid-1970s to 37 percent today.

[1]Reprint of an editorial article in *The Progressive*. Reprinted by permission of *The Progressive*, 54: 9–10. Ja '90. Copyright © 1990 The Progressive.

Hospitals have responded to the insurance shortfall by providing inadequate care for the poor, and by passing the costs of treating the uninsured on to patients fortunate enough to have coverage.

Medical costs continue to climb at a far faster rate than other prices. The United States spends more of its gross national product—11.2 per cent—on health care than any other nation, yet it trails in such indicators as longevity and infant mortality.

Against that background, it won't be long before Congress and even the Bush Administration will have to do *something*.

Chances are it will be the wrong thing.

Those conservatives who remain committed to privatization despite the fiascos of recent years are likely to push for a voucher system of some sort that would allow all citizens to buy health insurance through private insurers. The first problem with such a "solution"—as with similar schemes proposed for school reform—is that it would almost certainly be grossly underfunded, providing subsidies for the affluent but not enough to pay for decent coverage for the poor. And an immediate effect would be to compel workers to assume a greater portion of the costs of health insurance.

Some Congressional Democrats—notably Senator Edward M. Kennedy and Representative Henry Waxman—are backing a Federal version of the "Massachusetts plan" that would mandate a minimum level of employer-funded coverage, with limits on deductibles and on the premium share to be charged to employees. Provision would also be made for the gradual phase-in of the unemployed.

But the Kennedy-Waxman approach and the voucher plan share some fatal flaws. Both would perpetuate—and intensify—every significant defect in the current health-delivery system, including the inexorable pressure for higher and higher costs. Both would preserve the present irrational system of fee-for-service medicine, and both would perpetuate the power and enhance the profits of the insurance industry.

There is another approach that holds out higher hopes—an adaptation of the Canadian health-insurance system: All sums now paid for health-insurance premiums would go instead into a national health fund, which would be supplemented by appropriations from general revenues. Government would mandate minimum levels of care and would pay for most health services on a predetermined schedule of fees. Locally elected health boards would negotiate with hospitals on such decisions as the acquisition of costly technology.

Not the least virtue of such a system would be the elimination of private health insurance with its notorious mountains of paperwork. The Canadian experience suggests this innovation alone might save as much as $50 billion a year.

But the Canadian system is no cure-all. U.S. experience under Medicare and Medicaid demonstrates that some of the most difficult problems—and highest costs—are inherent in the practice of fee-for-service medicine. Physicians in private practice have little or no incentive to impose cost-control measures. And health-maintenance organizations have shown a proclivity to dump high-cost, high-risk patients.

In the long run, a humane, rational, and affordable health-care system will have to involve a greater say for health-care consumers. Citizens in a democracy are capable of making informed decisions on such questions as technological choice, the direction of research, and the curricular design of professional training. What's more, citizens can address the health-care issues that have always been slighted by the professionals: nutrition, occupational health and safety, environmental pollution, the effects of poverty on health.

A more democratic health-care system would make for a healthier citizenry—and a healthier democracy.

THE KILLER COST STALKING BUSINESS[2]

Imagine a recent Fortune 500 retiree named Fred, a prince of an employee over the years, but right now a corporate horror. Fred, 60, is covered by his company's health plan and has a life expectancy of 78; that's 18 years of health benefits. Young at heart, Fred has a new, 30-year-old wife who can expect to live to 80. She also comes under the company's health plan. So, gulp, does Fred Jr., 1 year old, whose coverage extends through the year he reaches 21. Add it up: 88 years of health benefits to be

[2]Reprint of an article by Carol J. Loomis, *Fortune* staff writer. Carol J. Loomis, *Fortune*, "© 1989 The Time Inc. Magazine Company. All rights reserved."

bestowed on a family that will be performing no work whatever for the company.

The example is obviously extreme. But when the subject is the promises that companies have made about health benefits, words of moderation mislead. All elements of this problem are enormous—the commitments, the expectations of employees, and potentially even their disappointments. Excruciatingly aware of what they have let themselves in for, companies are searching for roads of retreat. Some exist; most are tortuous.

Business is caught up, of course, in a national drama: The $550 billion the U.S. spent on health care last year amounted to nearly 11.5% of GNP, far more than in other industrialized countries. Costs are out of control, having risen since 1980 at a 10.5% annual rate. Many companies would kill to be so lucky. In 1987, General Motors' U.S. health care costs rose by 32%, to nearly $3 billion. Last year, says a consultant, the rise was again "horrendo."

The nation meanwhile equivocates about health costs, clamoring that they be contained yet demanding the easy availability of quality care. But no one wants to write the checks—neither the government, nor business, nor the patients.

The corporate obsession of the moment is retiree benefits, which around 70% of all large companies provide. In one way, these costs are no more than the tip of the iceberg: Typically, a corporation's health expenditures for active employees exceed those for retirees. But the actives *produce* and the retirees do not. Many, like Fred, are under 65 and prodigiously expensive to cover, since they do not yet qualify for Medicare. All those active employees, furthermore, are themselves marching toward retirement in cadence with a rapidly aging population. By the year 2020 or so the demographic profile of the entire nation is expected to match Florida's today: 18% of the population will be over 65.

These facts spell dollars, tons of them, and that reality should long ago have made managers fixated about their retiree costs. But in truth, most slumbered until shocked awake by accounting. Up to now, nearly all corporations have reported their retiree payments as the cash went out the door. But in the offing are new rules that would require companies to estimate all they will pay in the future, charge these obligations to their income statements, and recognize them as a liability on their balance sheets.

The obligations will be huge. One conservative estimate, by the Employee Benefit Research Institute, a nonpartisan, nonprofit organization in Washington, puts the present value of this liability, for all private employers, at $169 billion. Other estimates run as high as $2 trillion, not far below all the liabilities that nonfinancial corporations carry on their books. This vast discrepancy suggests the difficulty of pulling the problem into focus. But even the $169 billion figure implies that retiree health care costs will mangle many companies.

This problem also has a long tail, threatening to wrap itself around just about everybody in the country. Companies that provide retiree benefits feel compelled to attack this cost. But the moral and legal difficulties of cutting benefits for existing retirees have caused many companies to concentrate instead on reducing the benefits of their future retirees, a.k.a. their current employees. Many managements appear to detest this job—and all the other complexities of administering and policing health programs. A growing number yearn for some form of national health insurance to take over the task.

Many corporations edged into this bog during World War II, when wages were frozen and labor exacted health plans and other fringe benefits instead. Later, managements blithely extended like coverage to their non-unionized forces, retirees—and themselves. Health benefits have customarily been supremely egalitarian, linked to neither length of service nor salary.

That's one difference from pensions, among many. Most important, managements refused to index pensions to inflation. "Are you crazy?" they asked. "We can't afford that risk." But their health plans embraced indexing without ever using the word. Companies did not state their promises in terms of dollars—"We will give you X amounts to help defray your health costs"—but instead obligated themselves to cover their troops' medical bills, whatever these turned out to be.

They slipped into this awesome error partly because they viewed their health programs as short-term commitments subject to change, not long-term commitments like pensions. That thinking affected the financing of both. Wanting pension commitments to be solid, Washington required corporations to set aside funds to cover them at least partially, made contributions to these accounts tax deductible, and exempted their earnings from income tax. But the government did not prod employers to fund their health promises, nor did it shower them with tax incentives. As a result, only a few companies have done any funding at all. The rest pay as they go.

The pension vs. health differences—Arnold Schwarzenegger vs. Danny DeVito—extend to financial reporting. Corporations have long treated pensions as a form of deferred compensation. They thus account for these on an accrual basis, actuarially recognizing the cost of an employee's pension over his working life. But they did not bite this bullet with their retiree health plans. Instead, they reported their cash costs and let it go at that.

Into this haphazard world has now come the Financial Accounting Standards Board, saying, "These benefits, too, are a form of deferred compensation and thou shalt account for them in precisely that way." For retiree health benefits, then, it's out with pay-as-you-go reporting, in with accruals—which in virtually all cases will be higher.

The new rules will probably not apply until 1992 and may be modified as FASB exposes them to public and undoubtedly heated debate. But their shape can be anticipated. Corporations will first have to estimate future spending on health benefits for current and future retirees and all covered dependents. They must then discount these obligations to present value and begin charging them gradually to earnings.

These bookkeeping charges, while not affecting the cash companies pay for medical bills, will inflict big damage on that telltale report card, the income statement. The toll will be especially heavy for perhaps 15 years, as companies recognize liabilities built up in the past. After that, the charges will continue to hurt as they are accrued year after year. Meanwhile, each company's balance sheet will display the "debt" owed to retirees, present and future.

Estimating these obligations will be only slightly easier than making the sun rise in the West and set in the East. Take the example of Mrs. Fred. The company responsible for her must, in effect, estimate what her medical costs will be over 50 years, taking into account price inflation (What will a hip replacement cost in 2030?), the frequency with which she may use medical services (One hip or two?), and the impact of technology (Will they be using gold by then for hips?). And what to make of Medicare, the primary provider for those over 65, with business picking up the extras? Lately Medicare, by extending catastrophic coverage to citizens over 65, has assumed billions in costs formerly borne by business. But will this munificence last—through next year, much less for 49 more?

All these matters will, of course, be dealt with actuarially, though by what warm bodies is not clear. Right now, says Diana Scott, the FASB's project manager on this case, "there just aren't enough actuaries to do all the measurements." Some managements, in any event, will be seeking almost any excuse to forecast slow growth for health costs. Outside consultants say many of their clients are gravitating toward 6.5% to 8.5%, telling themselves that the current out-of-control rates just can't continue. The numbers, in short, are going to be lousy. Says Timothy Lucas, FASB's staff director: "We think they will still be better than what you get now, which is zero."

There are some estimates around and they are ugly. Harold Dankner, a Coopers & Lybrand consultant, has been working with 25 companies that are testing FASB's rules. For many of this crowd, he says, the retiree accrual costs are going to run three to six times the retiree pay-as-you-go costs. The worst dollar blows— no surprise—are due to fall on companies that have demographically mature groups of people to support.

Consider steelmaker LTV, a company mired in bankruptcy since 1986. Retiree health benefits did not exactly put it there. But they were always a rumbling issue, now erupted. Last fall, anticipating FASB's rules, LTV made a massive accrual for retiree health costs, charging $2.3 billion to earnings. That charge says nothing about LTV's ability to pay these costs, which is probably dubious, nor does it clean the company's accrual slate. LTV was simply stating that at its measurement date, year-end 1987, it was estimating $2.3 billion to be the present value of its obligation to its existing retirees and to its active employees for the years they had worked so far.

LTV took this step, says controller William P. Twomey, because the liability is "real" and should be out on the table in the bankruptcy proceedings. But he also acknowledges that LTV had a unique opportunity to get this cost behind it, since it was merely turning its negative net worth into a redder shade of red. Healthier companies, he suspects, could not tolerate the hit, since they would fear the impact on their net worth or on loan covenants.

The average company will indeed string its accruals out. One of the few talking publicly about their financial effects is Du Pont. Currently the company provides health coverage for 100,000 employees, 71,000 retirees or their survivors, and 275,000 dependents, for a total of 446,000 people. Last year, when pretax profits were $3.6 billion, Du Pont's out-of-pocket health costs for this multitude were around $410 million, of which some $180 million went to retirees. But, says A. Herbert Nehrling Jr., director of employee benefits, the company thinks that retiree accruals could be from two to four times the retiree payouts, depending on its assumptions about future health costs. In other words, the retiree expenses hitting Du Pont's 1988 income statement could hypothetically have been $360 million to $720 million, instead of $180 million.

A House committee heard a still spookier estimate last fall from an AT&T actuary, Michael Gulotta, who was representing a coalition of large corporations. He said the average company was facing accruals that would be four to five times its retiree pay-as-you-go expense. Say AT&T is this "average" company. In 1987 its payouts were $319 million, which means its hypothetical accruals would have been $1.3 billion to $1.6 billion. Those are thunderous figures in relation to the company's 1987 pretax profits of $3.2 billion.

Furthermore, comparisons to *pretax* profits themselves somewhat mislead, since that pair-off implies that these accruals will be costs that can be fully "tax effected"—that is, partially offset on a company's income statement by a reduced provision for taxes. But because of still other accounting rules going into effect for taxes, that will not always be so. Instead, large chunks of the accruals will, in the vernacular, fall straight to the bottom line.

The jolt to be delivered to the securities markets is hard to judge. Some of this heavy news has surely been discounted. Certain security analysts may also play down the new rules as mere bookkeeping that has little immediate relevance to cash flow. On the other hand, these charges could heighten the earnings disparities within industries—between an oldster like Inland Steel, say, and an upstart like Nucor, which does not offer retiree benefits.

The strongest reason for expecting jolts is the paucity of information on the retiree issue. Inexplicably, many companies have not focused at all on what FASB's rules mean for them. "I am staggered by this," says Donald G. McKinnon of the Mercer Meidinger Hansen benefits consulting firm. Some companies even lack a breakdown of today's costs for employees, retirees, and dependents. If companies are themselves so uninformed, it is hard to believe the market has anticipated all the news to come.

Many managements are on the prowl for ways to shrink this liability drastically. They carry a legal tool: The fine print in their health-benefit plans customarily notes the right of the employer to change these at will. But the legalities are in the ring with other powerful contenders, including employee relations and humane considerations.

Most important, the fine print will not provide managements with an escape from the essential moral dilemma, which concerns what the retiree is truly owed. Lawsuits brought over this issue have shown that most employees who were promised retiree health benefits never dreamed that they could be forced to bear sharply increased portions of the cost. They thought of their benefits as an entitlement. I worked, they say, therefore I earned.

There you have what Dallas L. Salisbury, president of the Employee Benefit Research Institute, calls the "social consciousness issue." Those not yet retired, Salisbury says, have time to adjust to changes in coverage: "They have time to work longer, time to save." They also have leverage, including the ability to strike or take another job. But, says Salisbury, "someone who is 78 and already has bad health problems does not have the option of finding new savings to pay health insurance premiums he never thought he would have to pay."

With an adjustment for age, he could almost have been talking about Charles Fletcher, 59, a retired distribution manager of American Forest Products, a California company taken private in 1981 by Kohlberg Kravis Roberts and that firm's most notable financial disaster. In 1983, as AFP cut back operations, Fletcher received $22,500 in severance pay and roundtripped $13,000 of it to AFP in exchange, so he thought, for lifetime health insurance for himself and his wife. Then in early 1988 he learned he had leukemia.

Three months later KKR sold AFP to Georgia-Pacific. AFP's retirees, including Fletcher, received notice from AFP that their health insurance would be terminated, but that they would each be paid $25,000 as compensation. Says Fletcher: "Most are older and come under Medicare, so they accepted. But for me, after taxes, that wouldn't cover one stay in the hospital." So he bitterly refused the $25,000 and is suing AFP and KKR. A lawyer for those companies says a clause in Fletcher's health plan permits the cancellation.

Fletcher joins a swarm of retirees who have sued to try to block their employers from modifying or terminating their health plans. Neither side has scored a legal knockout. "The law is in flux," says Timothy Ryan Jr., of Washington's Pierson Ball & Dowd law firm, which tends to represent the defense. No case has reached the Supreme Court. In district courts, the retirees have often won. Says Ryan: "We can eliminate juries, but we can't eliminate the typical 68-year-old judge. He doesn't like these cases at all." On appeal, where even 68-year-olds may apply the law strictly, judgments for the retirees have often been reversed, on grounds that the fine print is there and that they have no rights of contract.

Two lawsuits, with different verdicts, illuminate the texture of these cases. One action involved NLT Corp., a Nashville insurance company that had been acquired by another insurer, American General, which then sought to conform NLT's medical plan to its own. That meant NLT's retirees, who had been getting cost-free benefits, were hit for a share of the bill and they sued. The lead plaintiff—the kind you get in these cases—was a retired assistant secretary of NLT, Robert Musto, now 61, who had worked for the company 29 years.

The other action involved Bethlehem Steel and its retired managers, whose Blue Cross/Blue Shield policies had until 1985 been paid for by the company. When it then tried to shift some of the cost to the retirees, they sued. Their chief was a Bethlehem veteran of 31 years, Carroll G. "Gus" Heck. Now 63, he had been second-in-command at the company's Buffalo plant.

In the courtrooms where these two disputes were aired, the companies leaned on clauses in their plans permitting changes. In each instance, the retirees said they knew nothing of those clauses and had been orally promised cost-free benefits. The witnesses included managers who had done the promising, sometimes in "exit" interviews in which people set to retire were reminded of their cost-free coverage. NLT, especially, had trumpeted the virtues of its health plan. A retired vice president told about the spiel he delivered at meetings of district managers: "I would hit the fact that they were going to have paid-up medical insurance, hospitalization insurance at no cost to them or their wives after retirement."

In the NLT case, a Nashville district judge, only 54 years old in this instance, came down for the retirees. The promise of benefits, he said indignantly, is not "a mere gratuity, but rather a legal right derived from a unilateral contract." Wrong, said the appeals court, in a decision just handed down. Oral promises, the court said, were outweighed by NLT's written declaration that it could change its plan. Musto and crew are considering an appeal to the Supreme Court.

In the Bethlehem case, a Buffalo district judge, 67, also found for the retirees, 18,000 of them. He dismissed the we-reserve-the-right language in Bethlehem's medical plans as not meaning much, in part because it had been carelessly omitted from two summary documents. To claim the oral representations made at the exit interviews didn't matter, the judge said, would mean that Bethlehem had perpetrated "an enormous fraud" upon the plaintiffs.

Talking appeal, Bethlehem instead settled. In exchange for certain improvements in other benefits, the retirees accepted cost sharing in their Blue Cross/Blue Shield coverage. "It was a win-win situation," says Heck's lawyer, Richard Moot of Buffalo's Moot & Sprague. Seeming to agree, Bethlehem attorney Kathleen Mills says the company wanted to settle because it disliked being "in an adversarial position" with its own people. Says she: "We didn't see that something we forced down their throats through a court decree was going to make for peace, happiness, and wondrous living."

By now, many other company, inspecting this trunk of legal and moral problems, has decided its existing retirees must be treated gently. Or perhaps—you should pardon the expression—grandfathered while the employer moves on to cut the benefits of the next generation of retirees and the next.

Just to begin the exercise, a company must analyze its health plans from stem to stern. What has it promised and to what extent can it back away? The answers may drive it to nonegalitarian "solutions." Consultant McKinnon says many companies are thinking of borrowing a years-of-service concept from pensions. That is, the less time an employee has worked, the less he gets in company-paid benefits when he retires. Pillsbury has already adopted such an approach.

International Paper took a strikingly different tack in a plan it announced to its non-unionized employees in mid-1987. In a stair-step arrangement, the benefits of people who had retired before January 1, 1983, were grandfathered—that is, left untouched. Those who had retired since that date were required to pay increased premiums, while those headed for pasture in the future were told they would then be paying still more. And, last, in a bit of lightning that makes IP a retiree revolutionary, employees hired after October 1, 1987, would not have "subsidized" retirement coverage at all.

Yes, says William Fuller, an IP spokesman, that means the company won't pay a cent toward coverage—though it might, for example, help its employees get group rates. Since the company never provided retiree benefits for its hourly paid employees, says Fuller, "over time—a long time—we will eliminate this expense."

IP's plan also requires more premiums from retirees under 65 than from those over, which puts the company on the leading edge of a national trend. Early retirees can be a medical disaster. In the first place, some have retired early because they were sick. Second, sick or well, they are "time rich," able to hang out at the doctor's. Third, as they near 65, they may decide that the optional surgery they were considering should be done on their company's bill, before they have to tangle with Medicare's complexities.

So a corporate retiree of, say, 58 may run up medical bills about double those of the 58-year-old still working. Says Stephen C. Caulfield, a Mercer Meidinger consultant: "I tell my clients that if the only issue is health costs, then they don't want to push people into early retirement." But that is seldom the only issue. Restructurings and leveraged buyouts and even the old stuff, like 30-and-out retirement programs, keep putting these kids on the street.

Happily for IP, it could make its changes without bargaining with its unions. No labor leader has doubts about the value of health benefits and many have leaped to defend them from attack. In 1986, just after LTV went into bankruptcy, it tried to stop paying retiree health costs. The United Steelworkers promptly called a work stoppage—and LTV began paying again. That same year, the Communications Workers of America struck New York Telephone for nine days over issues that included the company's proposal that retirees and current employees start sharing the cost of their health coverage. That issue flamed the longest. "At its end, this strike was about health care, pure and simple," says George Kohl, the CWA's director of research. New York Tel did not get cost sharing.

This year, as contracts for all of the Bell companies come up once more, Kohl says the issues will be "one and two, job security and health care." At Nynex, parent of New York Tel, management is also brooding about health, partly because it dreads FASB's rules. Vice chairman William Burns says progress just has to be made on the union front: "All of us in corporate America know it's time for us to get this escalating cost monster under control."

He touches the heart of the problem. Companies may induce employees to smarten up their purchases of medical services or may even restrict their choice of suppliers. But there will still be a big bill on the plate and somebody—the company or the employee—must pay. Most corporations do not enjoy shifting costs to their employees. But in the interests of shareholders, they are naturally going about the job. The employees are just as naturally resisting. This conflict, sharp even now, is apt to turn brutal as FASB's rules bear down.

Some corporations have meanwhile been seeking help from Washington, campaigning for tax legislation that would permit employers to fund health benefit plans much as they do pension plans. Congress thinks the objective admirable, but not the means of getting there. Because this program would increase corporate tax deductions, it would cut federal revenues. In a read-my-lips era, cuts are not in the cards.

Instead, business may find the tables turned. There is talk of legislation that would cap employers' ability to deduct health costs—perhaps through a per capita limit. Would corporations fight such a measure? Many clearly would. But some might like to make such a cap an excuse for cutting benefits and escaping their "indexed," open-ended promises. Says consultant Caulfield: "I wouldn't be surprised to see industry sit on its hands on this one."

Amazingly, business seems even to be questioning its fundamental beliefs about health. The idea of government-run national health insurance available to all used to be almost universally despised by corporations. But now—behold the irony!—they seem to have experienced a certain conversion. Says Willis Goldbeck, head of the Washington Business Group on Health, a nonprofit organization backed primarily by big companies: "I find more and more businessmen are frustrated with this whole bloody effort. They see managing health as a forever deal. And they say, 'I'm not really in that business. Maybe some sort of national health insurance would make sense.'" Other health experts confirm Goldbeck's findings. There is a shift in the winds and it is not minor.

Nonetheless, the hard gusts of the next few years are apt to swirl mostly around retirees and FASB's rules and precisely who is to pay for a bill we can't pin to the mat. Want a useful suggestion? Tell your kid to become an actuary.

BITING THE INSURANCE BULLET[3]

Just a few years ago anyone proposing a national health-care program to a roomful of CEO's would have been met with hostile stares. A broad federal role in the health-care system was so out of favor that even advocates talked about it in hushed tones. It was considered too expensive, bureaucratic and, well, socialistic.

How quickly political fashions change: national health care is back in, and for the first time the idea is attracting support from business leaders. In April Chrysler chairman Lee Iacocca wrote that "maybe we should go to school on the national health care systems in Europe and Japan and design one for the United States." A "National Leadership Commission" brimming with business, medical and political leaders endorsed a major restructuring of the health-insurance system, including a guarantee of basic coverage for everyone. Even the Heritage Foundation, the conservative think tank, recently proposed a market-oriented health-care overhaul.

The reason for the growing corporate interest is simple: the cost of providing health care to employees has battered profits and strained competitiveness (NEWSWEEK, Jan. 30). In 1965 healthcare expenditures equaled 9 percent of corporate operating profits; in 1987 it was roughly 46 percent. The textile maker West Point-Pepperell, Inc., spends $35 million a year on health care, equal to the price of 8 million of its sheet-and-pillowcase sets. As of 1992 the impact of the books will become more dramatic as a new accounting rule requires firms to start reporting the costs of health coverage for future retirees.

Companies have absorbed much of the mounting tab themselves, but they're also asking employees to pay more. The divisiveness of that trend has become clear in the strikes against the Baby Bell phone companies. Nearly 200,000 phone-company workers went on strike, mostly over proposals to raise their medical payments. Last week Bell Atlantic seemed on the verge of settling (after it dropped a cost-sharing plan in favor of limits on where employees can seek care), but strikes at several other companies continued. Although union leaders acknowledge that

[3]Reprint of an article by Steven Waldman, *Newsweek* staff writer. Reprinted by permission from *Newsweek*, 114:46. Ag 28 '89. Copyright © 1989 by Newsweek.

health costs are hurting corporations, they say it's unfair to pass
the cost on to workers—and they, too, want a broader solution to
the crisis. "No one employer and no one union can solve this
at the bargaining table anymore," says the AFL-CIO's Karen Ig-
nagni. "The problem's just too big." When contracts were reached
at AT&T and Bethlehem Steel recently, they included labor-management agreements to lobby for a national attack on the health-
care problem.

While some unlikely allies have called for government action,
few agree on what that means. Proposals vary widely, and most
proponents prefer to talk about a "national approach" rather
than "national insurance." Many have looked at Canada's system,
which is privately run but government funded. The AFL-CIO has
proposed having Washington set minimum benefits and broad
cost limits, but letting states decide how to meet those goals. In
November of 1989 the AFL-CIO, which has backed national
health care for years, will launch a major campaign to drum up
support for its plan. The Leadership Commission recommended
creating a Universal Access Program, run by the state and funded
by employers and taxpayers, to help those not covered at work or
too poor to buy insurance.

STALLED REFORM

Doctors' groups contend that these approaches would erode
the quality of care. "Big business is saying, 'Let's let the government do it,' without realizing it would cause the slowing of technological innovation and make access to health care increasingly
difficult," says Dr. James Todd of the American Medical Association. He notes that in Canada, some advanced medical devices
aren't easily available and some surgery requires long waits.

So far Congress has been slow to respond to the growing
interest in a national approach. A bill sponsored by Sen. Edward
Kennedy that would mandate company insurance plans is stalled.
Meanwhile Congress is retreating from its last big health-care
reform, a Medicare surcharge for middle- and upper-class seniors
to fund a catastrophic-care program. Whether it's business or
government that takes the lead, any serious effort to roll back
costs will involve limiting medical fees and volume—and that's
bound to produce a political backlash from doctors and hospitals.
"In the real world we're years away from a government program," predicts Joseph Califano, a health consultant and former

cabinet official. Yet the coming political battles will be marked by one big change: the advocates of national health care will no longer just be Ted Kennedy liberals talking about the poor, but CEO's pointing to the bottom line.

THE CANADIAN MODEL[4]

With the increasing concern about deficiencies in health care delivery in the United States, and the Canadian experiment looming before you in the north, the question in the title of my talk was inevitable.

I was in private practice in Canada long before the advent of national health insurance there and continued to practice for some 15 years after its introduction. From this experience, I can draw certain conclusions. However, to discuss the question that is before us, I must begin by asking some questions of my own.

Constitutional and Political Issues

Because I acquired an honors degree in economics and political science before studying medicine, the first issue that came to my mind was whether it is constitutionally *possible* for the U.S. governments (state and/or federal) to institute (legally) a Canadian-style system.

Although you and I speak the same language, have much the same culture, are exposed to the same media influences, and spend a great deal of time in each other's countries, you must understand that the Canadian political structure, not to mention its national psyche, is very different from yours. Our parliamentary system, unlike your republican form, allows the man at the head of the party having simply a majority of seats in the House of Commons to do almost anything—and to get away with it. We have recently acquired a much-vaunted, so-called Charter of Rights. But unlike your Bill of Rights, it was so emasculated be-

[4]Reprint of an address before the 46th annual meeting of the Association of American Physicians and Surgeons by William E. Goodman, a Canadian physician. Reprinted by Permission of *Vital Speeches of the Day*, 56: 303–07. Nov 1 '90. © 1990 copyright by Vital Speeches of the Day.

fore being passed that it isn't worth the paper it's printed on. As for our psyches, the best way to compare them is to tell you that, while the key words in your Declaration of Independence are "life, liberty, and the pursuit of happiness," the key words in our constitution are "peace, order, and good government."

By and large, Canadians are middle-of-the-roaders who love security and hate to rock the boat. In contrast, Americans are a nation of protesters who tend to admire boat-rockers and self-made achievers. As Professor Russel Knight of the University of Western Ontario once said, "In the United States, everyone aspires to be an entrepreneur; in Canada, everyone wants to be a civil servant."

Notwithstanding these differences, both our governments learned long ago how to get around constitutional limitations and embarrassments. (Look at what's happened here since the passage of California's Proposition 13, and Washington's Gramm-Rudman Act.) In health care as in other matters, legislators have known since time immemorial that what could not be achieved by purely legislative measures could nonetheless be attained by fiscal arm-twisting—in other words, by bribery.

It's legal bribery, but still bribery, to make opponents an offer they can't refuse. That's what happened in Canada. Under our constitution, the federal government has virtually no powers in health matters. Yet, by taxing *everyone* across the country indiscriminately, but offering billions of dollars in grants to *only* those provinces that introduced a national health insured system of the federal government's choice, it finally forced all of them to participate.

From what I know of your constitutional setup, I believe it would be much more difficult, in legal terms, for your government to impose its will on a reluctant State, reluctant public, or reluctant profession. Nonetheless, I expect that the outcome for the U.S. health care system will ultimately be determined by the power of the dollar, not by ringing Jeffersonian statements.

Even if a Canadian-style model is constitutionally possible here, a second question arises: Would your doctors, your hospitals, your diagnostic laboratories, your insurance companies, your employers, and, most of all, your patients be prepared to pay the enormous cost involved? A recent U.S. public opinion poll showed that, although a majority of Americans would love access to such a Canadian-patterned system, only a very small minority were prepared to pay even $50 more a year. (So much for the validity of polls.)

And the cost is not measured solely in dollars. Much more important costs are a lack of access to health care personnel, institutions, diagnostic and therapeutic facilities; waits for essential services and surgery that run into years; and what I regret to have to refer to as the "lowest-common-denominator" quality of medical care. More about the last later.

Health Care Costs

It has been claimed that, according to the most recent statistics, Canadian medical care uses up about 8.6 percent of our gross national product, with full universal coverage, while U.S. health care consumes 12 percent of your GNP, even though some 35 million Americans reportedly have no health insurance at all. Without exploring possible reasons for the difference (e.g. leaving aside the fact that a lower percentage in Canada may actually mean a lower level of accessibility and quality), I find these figures highly suspect, based on previous experience with government statistics.

Our government's statisticians, like yours, are capable of enormous errors. Let me read you an Associated Press report from Washington, dated September 5, 1989:

> Chagrined economists watched in horror as the government made revision after revision last month in data on past performance that they use in their prognostications. The net result was that the economy was not nearly as weak during the spring as originally thought. Consumers spent at least double the pace first reported, employment growth was much stronger, and the overall economy, rather than limping along at an anemic annual growth rate of 1.7 percent from April through June, actually grew at a healthy 2.7 percent rate . . . The government's reports on factory orders and retail sales have been notoriously unreliable, and analysts have grown accustomed to looking at the figures with skepticism . . . The Labor Department's monthly employment report—generally considered one of the most accurate economic measurements— veered far off the mark earlier this year. Almost half the actual job growth in April, May, and June was missed in the original report.

As you all know, politicians and their minions are past masters in the art of disguising, manipulating, and fudging figures to their advantage, in addition to making presumably honest but gigantic errors. You will remember, to quote Mark Twain, that there are three kinds of lies: lies, damn lies, and statistics.

However, even if we accept the estimate of the percentages of our respective GNPs devoted to health care costs, the expense of health care in Canada is one of the major factors in a Canadian federal per capita debt and per capita annual deficit that is twice as bad as yours. As to provincial budgets, over a third of the revenue is already committed to health care, and the proportion is rising inexorably.

Notwithstanding these huge expenditures, the obvious deficiencies of the system are such that everyone—the public, the hospitals, the media, the doctors and nurses, the health economists, the budgetary experts, and even the government's own representatives speak incessantly about the crisis in our health care system. So what has gone wrong?

Apart from any political philosophy that you may espouse, be it free-enterprise or welfare-state, it's essential to realize that the basic and unalterable flaw in any system like the Canadian model is that, in economic terms, it is an open-ended scheme with closed-end funding. In other words, the potential demands are completely unrestricted, but the money to pay for them is not. It's like giving the public a no-dollar-limit, no-responsibility-for-payment medical credit card—an open invitation to unlimited abuse by both patients and doctors. Therein lies the politicians' dilemma: how to continue to buy votes with grandiose give-away schemes when it becomes evident that the money is running out. This is a generic problem, not confined to any one country or system of government. Its end result, no matter where practiced or how implemented, is always bankruptcy—unless major (and painful and politically very unpopular) changes are instituted in time, to the chagrin, disappointment, and detriment of the sick.

Canadian Vignettes: True Stories of "Universal Access"

How does one define the "Canadian model"? Let me paint you a few scenarios—all taken from the pages of Canadian newspapers and magazines, or from our broadcast media.

1. *You're sick and need access to some special diagnostic or therapeutic equipment,* but because of the constraints of government global

budgeting, your hospital (in this case the largest teaching hospital of the largest university faculty of medicine in Canada's largest city), can't afford it. Hospital administrators are having to go, hat in hand, begging for handouts from the general public or former patients, to buy the necessary machinery.

2. *You're sick and need to be admitted to your local community hospital but can't get in.* Notwithstanding the waiting list, many months long, of people with elective or urgent problems, the hospital has decided to close 12 percent of its beds—one in eight—taking them completely out of service because the government's refusal to provide adequate funding. At the same time, the hospital is legally prohibited from accepting any additional private payments that might have permitted it to continue in full operation.

3. *You're sick and need cardiac bypass surgery,* but the list of patients waiting for similar and sometimes more urgent surgery is so long that your hospital admission is postponed 11 times in the year before you finally come to surgery. Or you die of cardiac disease before your turn comes up. This has happened to many patients.

4. *You need an elective procedure like a lens implant or hip transplant.* Since your hospital has used up the annual allotment that the government allows, you are willing to pay the cost of the prosthesis yourself, rather than waiting ten months or a year until the hospital receives a new allotment. The answer is no. The government will not allow you to pay for your own procedure, and it is illegal for a doctor or hospital to participate in such a queue-jumping measure. (Interestingly enough, if you're an American or other foreigner who has seen fit to come to Canada at your own expense for the surgery, it *is* permissible.)

As Professor Arnold Aberman put it: "The monopoly on health care exercised by the government here is such that, if the government decides that *it* can't afford it, [Canadians] are not allowed [privately] to buy it." The only way for Canadians to get around this idiotic rule is to leave the country to go to the U.S.A. for the diagnostic or therapeutic modality they require.

5. *Your wife, your mother, your sister, or your daughter is asymptomatic but wants the reassurance of mammography or a Pap smear to rule out early breast or cervical cancer.* She has great difficulty arranging this because the government has decreed to the profession that these procedures are justified only in certain age or other risk groups and are not required more often than at certain specified intervals. The criteria used for making such determinations are epi-

demiological and have nothing to do with the well-being of the individual patient. To use their own euphemistic words, the government asks: "Is it cost-effective? Can it withstand economic appraisal?"

6. *You've had a sudden myocardial infarction* and your family wants your doctor to administer the drug TPA or APSAC immediately. They have read that it is more effective than the streptokinase currently used in most Canadian hospitals. The government or the hospital will not be willing to pay for the newer drug because it is much more expensive. And even if your family were willing to pay the extra cost themselves, permission for the doctor or hospital to use the drug might not be granted.

7. *You're a 37-year-old pregnant physician* in Vancouver and believe that you should have an amniocentesis to rule out genetic abnormalities in the fetus. By government edict, local doctors and hospitals cannot perform it, *even if you're willing to pay the total cost yourself*, unless you are over a certain age or have a specific history of genetic abnormalities. So you have to cross the border to Seattle if you wish to have the procedure, at considerable added expenditure of both time and money, *not* reimbursed by our government medical plan.

8. *You're a medical department head* in a university teaching hospital and need a certain complement of interns and residents for your department to function properly. But the government (which now pays the salaries of in-hospital personnel) says *no*. It thinks the country already has too many people in that specialty and besides, it can only afford half or two-thirds of the number you requested, so you'll have to make do with less. (In most cases, the government even refuses to allow house officers to work without pay, as some are willing to do in order to acquire necessary practical experience and academic credit).

9. *You're head of housekeeping* in one of the largest university teaching hospitals in Montreal and need a minimum number of workers to keep the wards clean and tidy. "Sorry," says the hospital administrator. The halls may be littered with old cartons, soft drink cans, and other garbage, but with its limited government budget, the hospital has to cut corners somewhere. There is not even sufficient money to pay for the nurses who are desperately required—and nurses are far more important than floor cleaners.

10. *You're the mayor* in a small, remote northern Ontario community. Your community hospital desperately needs money to upgrade its facilities, the only ones available for a very large but

sparsely populated region. In addition, you have great difficulty recruiting *any* doctors to settle and work in your rather less than desirable area. "That's your problem," say the provincial government authorities. They offer to give the hospital money only if, by refusing hospital privileges, you force any doctor working there to accept "capping," that is, maximum global annual payments.

11. *You're a family practitioner* and want to refer a patient with a particular problem to a particular specialist who has great expertise in that field. Unfortunately, he works in one of the hospitals in which doctors' incomes are capped annually, and he has already reached his maximum for the year. There being no incentive for him to work, since he would be earning absolutely nothing for the extra time and effort, he's off attending conferences, writing books, taking part in seminars, or even perhaps playing golf. Accordingly, your patient may have to wait eight to ten months for an appointment.

12. *You're a surgical specialist* doing cataract surgery or nasal surgery or arthroscopy. Tired of having a ten-month list of patients waiting for hospital facilities to become available, you decide to invest your own funds in your own first-class facility, thereby reducing your patients' wait to a couple of weeks. "Uh, uh," says the government bureaucrat. First, you will have to have a special license. Second, the bureaucrats will decide if and where and by whom such facilities may be set up, what procedures they will be permitted to perform, and how much they will be allowed to charge. Furthermore, government control is such that they have the legal authority to walk in at any time without a search warrant to review your pattern of operations and your patient files and to seize any records they like.

13. *Your child has been born prematurely* and needs highly specialized neonatal care to survive. Too bad. Although you live close to a large city with teaching hospitals associated with a university medical faculty, many of the beds in the critical neonatal service lie empty, out of service because of lack of funding. No functioning bed is available for your child in the entire city, and he has to be flown hundreds of miles to another city, or perhaps across the border to Buffalo or Detroit, where such beds are much more readily found. It's true that under these circumstances the provincial government will pay for most of the hospital costs involved, but neither you nor your wife will be reimbursed for trips back and forth to that location, for the necessary hotel accommodations, for the long-distance telephone calls, or for lost wages. And there is no

way to compensate a family for the emotional trauma of being hundreds of miles away from a loved one who is critically ill.

14. *You're a gourmet* who loves fatty French foods. You are approaching age 40 and have begun to worry about your cholesterol level. You ask your general practitioner or cardiologist to order the necessary laboratory tests. "Not necessary," says the health ministry—unless you're in a certain age group and demonstrate certain "identifying risk factors for coronary heart disease." Your GP isn't actually forbidden—yet—to order the tests, but he knows that if he does he'll be receiving telephone calls and letters from the ministry demanding that he justify his course of action. Net result: he probably won't order the test. As in most other areas of life, a threat, actual or implied, is sufficient for deterrence.

15. *You're an older physician* with a particular empathy for other old people and work 80 hour weeks visiting them at their homes or in nursing homes—calls that very few doctors are prepared to make nowadays and for which your patients are extremely grateful. But instead of receiving thanks from the health administrators, you are ordered to appear before a review committee. You've been "gouging the scheme," say the health police, costing the government thousands of dollars for "unnecessary visits"! You end up having to spend many hours of your precious time and many of your own dollars for a lawyer's services before you are completely exonerated by the quasi-judicial Medical Review Committee or the Health Disciplines Board.

16. *You're a specialist in private practice,* with a teaching appointment at a hospital affiliated with a medical school. Each year, the hospital, hit harder and harder by increasing costs due to technical advances and inflation, has been issuing more and more strident appeals to the medical staff for voluntary and sometimes not-so-voluntary donations to tide it over financial crises caused by government global budgets that often don't even cover the inflation rate. Under our system, hospital appointments, especially those in university hospitals, are very limited; and your right to admit your patients to that hospital depends entirely on such an appointment. Your unwillingness to contribute annual "donations" on a scale deemed adequate by the hospital authorities may bring a veiled threat of freezing—or even termination—of your academic appointment. It's a form of hidden but nonetheless compulsory additional taxation, enforced by what is now essentially an arm of the government—the hospital. To

quote the Dean of the Faculty of Health Sciences at one of our medical schools: "Governments across the country are in hot pursuit of cost containment . . . The medical schools have become increasingly dependent on service income generated by practicing academic clinicians." So you have now become a de facto hospital employee, generating income for your employer not only by admitting your patients but also, willingly or unwillingly, sharing your own piece-work income with it.

17. *You're a radiologist* specializing in mammography, for which the government has heretofore paid a professional reading fee of $17.50. Now, because the incidence of breast cancer in women is about one in ten, the female public and particularly the militant feminist organizations have started clamoring for regular universal screening for adult women. To placate them, the government agrees to set up radiographic screening centers. However, because of the added cost, radiologists are informed that *since they should be able to read 40 such films per hour, the payment rate per patient will be reduced*, in Ontario to $10 and in British Columbia to $5.00. The radiologists' society, insisting that adequate readings cannot be done at a rate of more than eight per hour, is appalled, and predicts that such superficial mass-produced readings will result in missed cases of cancer. No matter: the health minister is interested in epidemiological, not individual outcomes.

18. *You have just been diagnosed as having cancer* and require immediate radiation therapy. You live in Canada's largest city, boasting the two largest cancer centers in the country, but you are told that both have such long waiting lists that they're not accepting new patients. You are instructed to report to a cancer center in a distant Canadian city, or more likely to an American center, at an enormous cost in time and inconvenience, as well as money, to you and your family.

19. *You are a doctor in a small community* in one of Canada's smaller provinces. Since these areas have trouble attracting doctors at the best of times, you're working to death trying to provide services to your patients. Along comes a politically appointed "Commission on Selected Health Care Programs," to tell you that:

a) The supply and activities of doctors will have to be controlled to stop spiralling health care costs; b) Doctors admit too many people to hospitals, run too many unnecessary tests, write too many prescriptions, and prescribe expensive brand-name drugs [instead of] generics; c) Doctors should be penalized if their patients are admitted to hospitals and not operated on within 48 hours or, if operated, are not released within their expected length of stay.

So much for professional independence.

20. *You're a long-suffering Canadian taxpayer* and have been comparing notes with American friends. If an American works full-time for a full year, your friends complain, the total burden of taxes is so heavy that it consumes his entire income from January 1 to May 3. In other words, he has to work four months of the year for the government. To your horror, you discover that the comparable figures for a citizen of Ontario are January 1 to July 7th! A Canadian has to work over *six* months solely to satisfy government's constantly increasing demand for taxes.

21. *You are a family doctor,* and a patient with a serious but not immediately life-threatening illness is furious when he's told that he'll have to wait three to six months for an appointment to see a particular specialist and six to 18 months for urgent hospitalization. What advice do you give him? The answer is obviously to buy a health insurance policy offered to Canadians by U.S. insurance companies for treatment in the U.S. Since 90 percent of Canadians live within 100 miles of the American border, it's no great problem for them to drive to Boston, Albany, Buffalo, Detroit, Cleveland, Seattle, or a dozen other border cities.

Other Problems

I'm sorry to overwhelm you with such a lengthy litany of horrors, but we see, hear, and read such repeated references in your media to the marvels of the Canadian model that I felt it essential you should know some of the warts on this much-touted scheme. I've restricted myself to the problems arising from the financial absurdity of the system. But there are many others, equally important: the total loss of medical confidentiality; the loss of morale and dedication among medical personnel; the loss of health care workers by emigration, change of vocation, or early retirement; the massive intrusion by the bureaucracy into the doctor-patient relationship; the civil servantization and inevitable unionization of the medical profession; and so on. It would take five more lectures of this length to describe in detail all the pernicious ramifications of socialized medicine, Canadian style.

Will the Canadian System Be Transplanted?

Returning to the questions that I posed earlier: Could the U.S. government introduce a scheme like the Canadian one in this country, regardless of constitutional niceties? The answer is clearly yes. What the politicians can't do by purely legislative means, they will accomplish by financial coercion.

Will the U.S. accept it? For the public, the answer, I'm sorry to say, is yes—overwhelmingly and gladly. They'd love it, because 95 percent of them won't understand its long-term effects on their lives, their liberties, their access to first-class medical care, or even on their pocketbooks. All they would know is that they had to pay nothing out of pocket at the time and place of actual medical service, at least initially. The vast majority of Canadians had and still have similar difficulties in associating "free" benefits on one hand with massive increases in taxes, public debt, and inflation on the other. Canadians still do not understand that their rapidly decreasing access to first-class medical care is an inevitable consequence of these "benefits."

As to industry, unionized facilities such as Lee Iacocca's Chrysler Corporation and many members of the National Association of Manufacturers have already indicated that they would welcome Canadian-style medicine with open arms. Why not? It would allow them to foist onto the general taxpayer most of the cost of their present employee health plans. In the long run, they'll rue the day, but industry tends to concentrate on the needs and stresses of the moment without much concern for the long-range perspective.

As to physicians, most would, sad to say, also approve of the Canadian scheme—whether because of inertia, as in older doctors; or out of a fatalistic resignation to what many consider inevitable; or because they realize, from the experience of the medical profession after introduction of national health insurance in other countries, that they will earn far *more* money than at present, at least for the first few years; or because they actually welcome increasing government intervention out of philosophical convictions, possibly due to having grown up in an increasingly welfare-state, do-gooder environment. Whatever the cause, I predict that over 80 percent of your doctors would raise no significant objection to national health insurance. Some will grumble and scream; some will threaten and issue bulletins; some may even withdraw services temporarily. But eventually, especially if significant financial or other penalties are involved, the rush to join the bandwagon will be overwhelming. This has been the experience in nations all over the world, and I see no reason to believe that U.S. response will be different. You have already seen a portent of this in the alacrity with which American doctors have joined HMOs or accepted Medicare assignment, even where it was not mandatory.

As to health-related industries, their acceptance will at first be grudging because of the perceived governmental regulation. However, I would remind you of American economics Nobel laureate George Stigler's famous pronouncement that regulation usually ends up benefiting those being regulated. Consider the billions of dollars earned by the defense industries under government regulation. Who minds a little supervision when the supervisors will approve a $650 toilet seat?

Would the System Lead to Bankruptcy?

The U.S. is still better off financially than Canada. But that situation will not long survive the introduction of a few of our open-ended social welfare schemes like national health insurance. Soon, the U.S., like Canada, would start lowering medical and institutional standards and reducing access to care. However, it takes a number of years for this to happen. In the meantime, the politician who fostered and promoted the system will be collecting votes, and the massively increased bureaucracy will have acquired a vested interest in maintaining and expanding the play. It took almost 20 years after the introduction of socialized medicine in Ontario for the politicians to grudgingly acknowledge, as our Minister of Health did last year, that "health care spending is on a collision course with economic realities." Yet any first-year economics student could have predicted, 20 years ago, exactly what would happen.

Conclusions

Let me give you the short answer to the question posed in the title of this address. If you define "could the Canadian model work here?" to mean "would it improve quality and accessibility of health care for a majority of Americans? my answer is yes—but only temporarily. Your citizens, like ours, will experience only briefly the medical Utopia that they have been promised, and at an enormous and eventually unbearable cost. Given your government's already astronomical deficits, I would guess that the time before imminent financial collapse would be much shorter than in Canada—perhaps five years.

The crux of the problem in any national health insurance program like the Canadian one is the large and ever-increasing gap between politicians' extravagant promises, public expectations arising from those promises, and cruel financial reality. The reality, sad as it may seem, is that not even you, the richest country in the world can afford everything for everybody for very long.

It's a pretty dismal picture, isn't it? Yet, if you think about it, this is a hopeful circumstance for AAPS. You and others who share your beliefs have a long and bitter struggle ahead, with many disappointments. But I'm convinced that in the long run, you'll prevail. You'll win, not only because you have the courage of your convictions and the will to continue fighting, but because the Canadian-style edifice that your opponents are in the process of constructing is built on sand.

BIBLIOGRAPHY

An asterisk (*) preceding a reference indicates that the material or part of it has been reprinted in this book.

BOOKS AND PAMPHLETS

Amara, Roy, Morrison, J. Ian, and Schmid, Gregory. Looking ahead in American health care. McGraw-Hill. '88.

Andreopoulus, Spyros. National health insurance: can we learn from Canada? Krieger. '87.

Barondess, Jeremiah, Rogers, David, and Lohr, Kathleen. Care of the elderly patient, policy issues and research opportunities. National Academy Press. '89.

Bender, David L. and Leone, Bruno, eds. The health care crisis: opposing viewpoints. Greenhaven Press. '89.

Bennett, Addison C. Maximizing quality performance in health care facilities. Aspen. '89.

Bergthold, Linda. Purchasing power in health: business, the state, and health care politics. Rutgers University Press. '90.

Berman, Melissa A. A harder look at health care costs. Conference Board. '88.

Blank, Robert. Rationing medicine. Columbia University Press. '88.

Butler, Stuart M. and Haislmer, Edmund F. A national health care system for America. Heritage Foundation. '89.

Callahan, David. What kind of life: the limits of medical progress. Simon & Schuster. '90.

Caro, Francis and Blank, Arthur. Quality impact of home care for the elderly. Haworth Press. '89.

Chernoff, Ronni and Lipschitz, David. Health promotion and disease prevention in the elderly. Raven Press. '88.

Churchill, Larry R. Rationing health care in America: perceptions and principles of justice. University of Notre Dame Press. '87.

Coile, Russell C. The new medicine: reshaping medical practice and health care management. Aspen. '90.

Davis, Karen. Health care cost containment. Johns Hopkins University Press. '90.

Dougherty, Charles J. American health care: realities, rights, and reforms. Oxford University Press. '90.

Eisdorfer, Carl, Kessler, David, and Spector, Abby. Caring for the elderly: reshaping health policy. Johns Hopkins University Press. '89.

Frech, H. W., ed. Health care in America: the political economy of hospitals and health insurance. Pacific Institute for Public Policy. '88.

Ginzberg, Eli. The medical triangle: physicians, politicians, and the public. Harvard University Press. '90.

Goldstein, Marion. Family involvement in the treatment of the frail elderly. American Psychiatric Press. '89.

Goodman, John C. and Musgrave, Gerald L. Health care after retirement. National Center for Policy Analysis. '89.

Hiatt, Howard H. America's health in the balance: choice or chance? Harper & Row. '87.

Horn, Barbara J. Facilitating self care practices in the elderly. Haworth Press. '90.

Inlander, Charles B., Levin, Lowells, and Weiner, Ed. Medicine on trial: the appalling story of ineptitude, malfeasance, neglect, and arrogance. Prentice Hall. '88.

Jones, Rochelle. The supermeds: how the big business of medicine is endangering our health care. Scribner. '88.

Jones, Jr., Woodrow and Rice, Mitchell F. Health care issues in Black America: policies, problems, and prospects. Greenwood Press. '87.

Kapp, Marshall B. Legal aspects of health care for the elderly: an annotated bibliography. Greenwood Press. '88.

Kellogg Foundation. Stemming the rising costs of medical care. The Foundation. '88.

Killeffer, Eloise and Bennett, Ruth. Successful models of community long term care services for the elderly. Haworth Press. '90.

Kilner, John F. Who lives? who dies? ethical criteria in patient selection. Yale University Press. '90.

Manning, Willard G. Health insurance and the demand for medical care. Rand. '88.

Matthews, Joseph and Berman, Dorothy. Social Security, medicare, and pensions. Nolo Press. '90.

McCue, Jack D., ed. The medical cost-containment crisis: fears, opinions, and facts. Health Administration Press Perspectives. '89.

McKenzie, Nancy F., ed. The crisis in health care. Meridian. '90.

_____ Painful choices: research and essays on health care. Transaction Publishers. '89.

Melhado, Evan, Feinberg, Walter, and Swartz, Harold, eds. Money, power, and health care. Health Administration Press. '88.

Melville, Keith. Health care for the elderly: moral dilemmas, mortal choice. Domestic Policy Association. '88.

Mooney, Gavin and McGuire, Alistair. Medical ethics and economics in health care. Oxford University Press. '88.

Morris, Jonas. Searching for a cure: national health policy from Roosevelt to Bush. Seven Locks Press. '90.

Mulvihill, James E. Health care for the elderly. Association of Academic Health Centers. '88.

National Leadership Commission on Health Care. For the health of a nation: a shared responsibility. Health Administration Press. '89.

Pearman, William and Starr, Philip. Medicare: a handbook on the history and issues of health care services for the elderly. Garland. '88.

Pegels, C. Carl. Health care and the older citizen: economic, demographic, and financial aspects. Aspen. '88.

Peterson, Marilyn and White, Diana. Health care of the elderly: an information sourcebook. Sage. '89.

Qureshi, Hazel and Walker, Alan. The caring relationship: elderly people and their families. Temple University Press. '89.

Rowland, Diane. Help at home: long-term care assistance for impaired elderly people. Commonwealth Fund Commission on Elderly People Living Alone. '89.

Scheffler, Richard M. and Andrews, Neil C., eds. Cancer care and cost: DRGs and beyond. Health Administration Press Perspectives. '89.

Shaffer, Franklin A. and Beyers, Marjorie. DRGs, nursing, and health care. W. B. Saunders. '88.

Strosberg, Martin, Fein, Alan, and Carroll, James, eds. Rationing of medical care for the critically ill. Brookings Institution. '89.

Swartz, Katherine. The medically uninsured. University Press of America. '89.

Szumi, Bonnie, ed. The health crisis: opposing viewpoints. Greenhaven Press. '89.

U. S. Congress. Hearings before the Subcommittee on Education and Health of the Joint Economic Committee. The future of health care in America. U. S. Government Printing Office. '89.

U. S. Congress. Hearing before the Pepper Commission. Assessing the affordability of private long-term care insurance. U.S. Government Printing Office. '90.

U. S. Congress. Hearing before the Pepper Commission. Options in access to health care. U. S. Government Printing Office. '90.

U. S. Congress. Report by the Chairman of the Select Committee on Aging. Emptying the elderly's pocketbook—growing impact of rising health care costs. U. S. Government Printing Office. '90.

U. S. Congress. Hearing before the Select Committee on Aging. Building an American health care system: journey toward a healthy America. U. S. Government Printing Office. '90.

U. S. Congress. Report by the Chairman of the Select Committee on Aging. Medicare coverage of catastrophic health care costs: what do seniors need, and what do seniors want? U. S. Government Printing Office. '90.

U. S. Congress. Subcommittee on Labor-Management Relations. Hearings on the growing crisis in health care. U. S. Government Printing Office. '90.

U. S. Congress. Hearings of the Committee on Labor and Human Resources. The American health care crisis: a view from four communities. U. S. Government Printing Office. '90.

U. S. Congress. Hearing before the Subcommittee on Housing and Consumer Interests. The future of health care for seniors: where do we go from here? U. S. Government Printing Office. '90.

U. S. Congress. Hearing before the Select Committee on Children, Youth, and Families. The changing face of health care: the movement toward universal access. U. S. Government Printing Office. '90.

U. S. Department of the Treasury. Financing health and long-term care: report to the President and to the Congress. U. S. Government Printing Office. '90.

Walsh, John, Tsukuda, Ruth, and Miller, Judy. Management of the frail elderly by the health care team. W. H. Green. '89.

Wiest, Walter E. Health care and its costs: a challenge for the church. University Press of America. '88.

Williams, Sandra and Allen, Isobel. Health care for single homeless people. Policy Studies Institute. '89.

ADDITIONAL PERIODICAL ARTICLES WITH ABSTRACTS

For those who wish to read more widely on the subject of health care, this section contains abstracts of additional articles that bear on the topic. Readers who require a comprehensive list of materials are advised to consult the *Readers' Guide to Periodical Literature* and other Wilson indexes.

Health care costs take a turn for the worse (employer-union cooperation). Joan O'C. Hamilton, *Business Week* 120 O 31 '88

A new wave of health care inflation threatens to undermine the progress that unions and employers have made in cutting health care costs without reducing benefits. For a while, tactics such as second opinions and outpatient clinics helped check rising prices, but the medical establishment has discovered ways to counter the new controls. The government's efforts at controlling medical costs have also proved ineffective. As a result, unionized companies may soon shift more of the cost to workers, and many nonunion employees may also be expected to pay more for their health insurance. Employers and unions are strengthening their efforts to impose controls, but the cost of health care is not expected to decline in the near future.

High-tech health care: who will pay? Joan O'C. Hamilton, Emily T. Smith, and Susan B. Garland, *Business Week* 74-6+ F 6 '89

New medical technologies hold the promise of saving many lives, but their high cost has prompted a debate over who will pay for them and who will have access to them. Individuals and businesses are already struggling to meet the rising costs of traditional health care, and an increasing number of insurance providers are refusing to cover high-tech treatment. On the other hand, Americans feel entitled to the best possible medical care. Several proposals have been advanced for rationing high-tech care, such as placing limits on treatment of elderly patients or limiting care for patients whose lifestyles have brought about their illnesses. Some of the experts who evaluate the safety and effectiveness of new technologies want to judge them on the basis of cost as well. When state and federal legislators have tried to implement this strategy, however, they have been criticized by those who believe that it measures the value of life by the bottom line.

Ouch! The squeeze on your health benefits (cover story) *Business Week* 110-13+ N 20 '89

A cover story discusses corporate America's efforts to control the escalating costs of worker health care benefits. the nation's medical tab comes to an annual $541 billion, or 11 percent of its total economic output, the largest percentage of any industrialized country. Corporations are implementing a variety of experimental plans to reduce their health care bills. They have tried increasing workers' share of health care costs, group medical plans, more outpatient care, preferred provider organizations, preapproval of many hospital procedures, and fitness programs that promise to reduce medical bills in the long term.

Health care costs: trying to cool the fever: insurers and companies are coming up with new containment ideas Susan B. Garland, *Business Week* 47 My 21 '90

The insurance industry is pushing a number of state bills that would allow insurers to sell policies to small employers that do not include such state-mandated benefits as mammography screening, alcoholism treatment, or mental health services. Insurers claim that the cost of such benefits discourages many small employers from offering any coverage at all. Health care providers and advocates for the disadvantaged contend, however, that mandates are only a minor reason for rising health care costs and that dropping them will cause health care to suffer.:BRDG90024685

The health care quagmire (cover story) Edmund F. Haislmaier, *Consumers' Research Magazine* 72:10–16 S '89

An article excerpted from A National Health System for America. Growing concern over the escalating costs of and limited access to the U.S. health care system has led lawmakers and private employers to explore ways of reducing costs and closing the gaps in coverage. An examination of the history of health care in the United States shows an emphasis on employer-paid plans, front-end and acute-care coverage, and third-party insurance payments, with virtually no incentives for consumers to question the necessity of medical procedures or for providers to lower costs. The primary thrust of health care legislation and regulation since the 1970s has been to control costs, but little has been done to encourage health care providers to become more efficient and innovative. Unless basic structural deficiencies are rectified to reward consumers and providers for their cost consciousness, any attempt to solve individual health care problems will fail.

Live and let die Linda Marsa, *Omni* (New York, N.Y.) 11:40–2 S '89

Part of a cover story on social and environmental problems. Around the world, the state of health care is bleak. Medical care in some Third World countries has improved, but practices remain outdated, sanitation is poor, and malnutrition is common. Great Britain's system of socialized medicine is beset by crises, and even Canada's government-funded national health insurance system, one of the bright spots in the picture, is experiencing bottlenecks and rising costs. In America, the nation's medical bill is rising at two and a half times the inflation rate, and critics charge that Americans aren't getting much for their money. More than 37 million Americans are without health insurance, and another 15 million have inadequate coverage. Experts warn that fundamental changes must be made to avoid disaster.

Money, medicine and homelessness (Institute of Medicine report; special section) *Society* 26:4–23 My/Je '89

A special section examines health care and the homeless. Ten members of the Institute of Medicine's Committee on Health Care for Homeless People endorse the committee's report Homelessness, Health and Human Needs and make a supplementary statement that homelessness causes or exacerbates health problems that include hypothermia, lead poisoning, battery, rape, and AIDS. Unable to pay for health care, the homeless often do not receive it. Only a comprehensive, long-term strategy for eliminating homelessness will permanently improve this group's health. Decent housing is every American's right, and the federal government has an obligation to make it affordable by increasing the minimum wage, entitlement benefits, and funds for housing programs. Other articles discuss the costs of housing, dissension among scientists, the context of homelessness, and the economic, clinical, and political needs of the homeless.

Rationing medical care John Elson, *Time* 133:84+ My 15 '89

A growing number of experts believe that the United States is financially unable to provide unlimited medical treatment for all its citizens and that it must begin rationing health care. Most Americans find this idea morally repugnant, but a survey found that only one in ten people would accept a $125 tax increase to support nationwide insurance for catastrophic illness. Experts in favor of medical rationing point out that it is not really new. Many doctors admit, for example, that applicants for many high-tech operations are selected on the basis of their ability to pay. Several areas of the country are now taking more drastic measures. Oregon's senate has passed a bill that would extend Medicaid coverage to 86,000 people not currently insured but would limit the care they could expect. In California's Alameda County, a professional ethicist and a committee of medical experts will decide what medical services will be made available to the uninsured poor.

Insurance fraud hurts everybody Richard E. Earley, *USA Today* (Periodical) 119:62–4 Jl '90

Fraudulent insurance claims hurt honest people by inflating costs and changing the assumptions that insurance firms use to determine rates. The Insurance Information Institute estimates that false claims cost the public as much as $15 billion a year. Insurance fraud includes staged auto accidents, inflated repair costs, vehicles abandoned by their owners and reported stolen, false medical charges, contrived slip-and-fall accidents, and arson. Such crimes are not limited to any geographic region or segment of society, but they are most common in areas experiencing economic problems. Most are perpetrated by repeat offenders. Insurance companies have begun to fight fraud by establishing special investigative units, training claims representatives to recognize signs of fraud, and exchanging information with government agencies, health care professionals, and other insurance firms. BRDG90035064

Rent-a-docs Ellen Paris, *Forbes* 142:160+ N 28 '88

Small but growing numbers of doctors are giving up private practice to become temporary doctors who fill in at such medical treatment centers as hospitals and urgent-care clinics. These doctors usually receive a flat fee that varies from $225 to $300 a day for an internist to approximately $500 a day for an anesthesiologist. They are paid by the agency that places them. The agency usually also pays licensing fees, malpractice insurance premiums, and transportation. The medical service hiring the temporary doctor most often pays the housing costs. A conservative estimate places the number of temporary doctors at about 5,000, compared with 2,500 two years ago. Physicians decide to become temporary doctors for various reasons. Some want time off and freedom from the hassles of running a private practice, some want exposure to various medical fields, and others are nearing retirement and are fed up with the cost of malpractice insurance.

The bottom line is society loses (privatization) Mimi Abramovitz, *The Nation* 245: 410–12 O 17 '87

The increasing privatization of health care in the United States has led to the sacrifice of sound and equitable patient care. Since the 1970s, new corporate tax breaks, the exemption of health-care institutions from antitrust provisions, and the shaky financial state of many hospitals and nursing homes have led to the growth of large health-care chains. These for-profit institutions make a lot of money: by the 1980s the 38 major investor-owned chains had profit margins of 15 to 30 percent. Several recent studies have found that for-profit hospitals provide more costly care than voluntary and public hospitals. They resort to staff cutbacks, technological displacement, and union busting to bring down labor costs. When hospitals fail to bring in enough revenue, management does not hesitate to close service units or entire facilities. For-profit hospitals also prefer insured patients with uncomplicated diagnoses to those who are more medically and financially needy.

Cancer comes home Steve Fishman, *The New York Times* Magazine 70–1 Je 11 '89

Primarily as a result of the federal government's pressure on hospitals to cut costs, an increasing number of cancer patients are being given treatment at home. Although physicians still manage care from a hospital or office, day-to-day treatment has become the responsibility of the patient, even when the treatment involves high technology. The trend is also partially attributable to the fact that some 50 percent of patients will survive at least five years after being diagnosed with cancer, compared to only 33 percent 20 years ago. Although home care agencies and community health nurses provide help in these situations, it is not always easy for cancer patients and their families to cope with the requirements of home care, and family members often need outside help to meet the emotional demands of the arrangement.

Control of misconduct in medicine *Society* 25:5–6 My/Je '88

A perceived failure of the medical profession to police itself has stimulated legislative action intended to increase the responsibilities of individual medical practitioners and medical organizations to report medical malpractice. The federal government and many states have enacted or strengthened laws governing the reporting of malpractice or are considering doing so. Most of these laws assure immunity to those who make good faith reports to professional review boards. Many of the new laws require hospitals to report to state licensing authorities when they revoke or limit a health-care professional's privileges. Some of the laws will make it more difficult for incompetent doctors to move their practices from state to state. The trend in medical legislation could encourage changes in legislation affecting other professions.

It's fever time for doctors Clemens P. Work, *U.S. News & World Report* 102:44–6 Ja 26 '87

Economic pressures are causing what one doctor calls a shakeout among physicians. The glut of new doctors is leveling income increases, and business costs are traveling upward. At the same time that government and industry are pushing doctors to contain costs, consumer advocates are watching to make sure that doctors don't shortchange their patients. Health-maintenance organizations, walk-in clinics, and other types of corporate health care are forcing doctors to practice in unfamiliar surroundings. Moreover, doctors are upset at their gradual loss of prestige and authority. Many have opted for a group practice rather than a private one to reduce costs, cover for each other, and better negotiate with insurers. Others, particularly older doctors are leaving the medical field altogether. The changing times, however, have opened some new administrative opportunities or physicians.

There's no place like home Steven Findlay, *U.S. News & World Report* 104:68–70 Ja 25 '88

Health care in the home has become a popular alternative to hospital care, but families must choose assistance services carefully. Health professionals say that patients recuperate more quickly at home because of the psychological boost that the familiar environment provides. Some home-health services are one-half to one-third less expensive than comparable hospital care, thanks in part to the advent of transportable health equipment. Home health care is not without problems, however. In many regions, patients must now choose among dozens, or even hundreds, of agencies that vary greatly in costs and quality of care. In about one-third of the states, careful selection is a must because home-care services are not licensed. In addition, many insurance policies do not cover home care. Legislation that would provide federal assistance for home care of Medicare patients is awaiting congressional approval. Tips on selecting services are provided.

Is Medicare a terminal case? Susan B. Garland, *Business Week* 28 F 5 '90

Medicare's Hospital Insurance Trust Fund is likely to go bankrupt by 2005, according to the fund's trustees. Because of increasing health care costs and the graying of the country's population, Medicare, which pays for hospital and short nursing-home stays for the elderly, is expected to start paying out more than it takes in by 1998. Lawmakers are not eager to raise taxes for current workers or to cut benefits for current retirees, however. One remedy, promoted by former Social Security commissioner Robert M. Ball, would be to transfer part of the Social Security tax revenue to Medicare, thus extending the program until 2020. The Advisory Council on Social Security plans to investigate other ways to preserve government retirement programs.

Long-term care's staggering cost Louise Crooks, *Modern Maturity* 31:14–15 O/N '88

The Medicare Catastrophic Coverage Act, which is to take effect on January 1, 1989, is an important step toward reducing the costs of long-term health care, although it does not provide comprehensive coverage for the especially devastating costs of long-term nursing home care. The law will limit Medicare beneficiaries' expenses for huge hospital and doctors' bills and for outpatient prescription drug bills of over $600 a year. It will also offer some relief for caregivers with elderly or disabled family members at home, and spouses of nursing home residents will no longer be forced into abject poverty in order to qualify for Medicaid assistance.

Insuring against the cruel cost of long-term care Lani Luciano, *Money* 17:97–9 Ap '88

A major financial risk for older people is the high cost of long-term care for those who can no longer look after themselves. On the average, nursing homes cost about $24,000 per year, and Medicare does not cover all nursing-home stays. The best alternative is a retirement residence called a life-care community, which provides medical and personal care for the elderly in or out of a nursing home. Such residences usually have entrance fees of at least $20,000, however. Another alternative is a specialized health maintenance organization with long-term-care service. Most people's only option is buying a long-term-care insurance policy. The premium is likely to cost more than $1,000 per year, but even so, people over 50 should not put off buying such a policy.

Catastrophic follies (Medicare surcharge) Phillip Longman, *The New Republic* 201:16–18 Ag 21 '89

The Medicare Catastrophic Coverage Act passed by wide margins in June 1988, but there is now talk of repealing it. The Gray Lobby was appalled from the start by the White House's insistence that the program be funded by the elderly. In addition, some feared that the catastrophic hospital coverage would preempt the more coveted benefit of long-term nursing home care. By the time Congress finished amending the bill, it offered free hospital and physician care above $2,000 a year as well as a range of other benefits, all of which were to be paid for by a 15 percent income tax surtax on Medicare participants who are relatively affluent. It is true that the catastrophic program is a bad deal for the affluent elderly, but the other benefits provide compensatory gains.

Financing long-term care Jane Bryant Quinn, *Newsweek* 113:52 Ja 30 '89

Part of a cover story on the soaring cost of health care. Long-term health care for elder Americans, whether in the form of home care services or nursing homes, is tremendously expensive. Under the current system, seniors are responsible for their own care until their income and assets are nearly exhausted, at which point Medicaid covers their bills. Many elderly object to the depletion of their savings, as they would like to be able to leave more money to their children. Many seniors are doing this by giving their property to their children while they are still alive, claiming poverty, and turning to the taxpayers to finance their care. A number of proposals to help underwrite the burden of long-term care are being circulated, including a comprehensive federal program, a federal home health program, expanded private insurance, and a blend of private and government-sponsored coverage.

A victory for the haves? (Congress votes to trim catastrophic health care due to uproar over income tax surcharge) Eleanor Clift, *Newsweek* 114:38 O 16 '89

Congress has voted to repeal the Medicare Catastrophic Coverage Act of 1988 in the wake of a well-orchestrated direct mail campaign by retirees angry about the extra taxes the program imposed on them. Under the provisions of the program, all seniors would have paid a $4 monthly fee. Those with federal income-tax liabilities over $150 a year would have also paid a controversial 15 percent surcharge to help pick up the tab for poorer seniors. The top surcharge of $800 would have applied to only the wealthiest 5 percent of the elderly, but a key lobbying group called the National Committee to Preserve Social Security and Medicare apparently misled many retirees into thinking that it applied to them. The result of the repeal is that most of the nation's elderly will be faced with shrinking coverage at a time of escalating costs.

The short life of catastrophic care (repeal spurs medigap policies) Steven Findlay, *U.S. News & World Report* 107:72–3 D 11 '89

The recent congressional repeal of the catastrophic care law will force some elderly citizens to make difficult choices. With the repeal of the law, which greatly expanded benefits for 33 million elderly and disabled people, Medicare coverage will revert to nearly its former status. The only provision of the catastrophic care bill to be preserved is a Medicaid change that allows the spouse of someone entering a nursing home to keep $786 a month in income and $12,000 in assets. To fill the gaps left by the repeal, private insurance companies that sell health policies that supplement Medicare, called Medigap policies, are required by law to adjust their plans to take the loss of coverage into account. For individuals who bought new Medigap policies over the past year, insurers will likely offer a range of coverage options.

The catastrophic health care fiasco John L. Hess, *The Nation* 250:698–700+ My 21 '90

America's elderly have been unfairly attacked for their role in the demise of the Catastrophic Medicare Act of 1988. The bill, an unexpected extension of Medicare in an era of cutbacks in social programs, was passed overwhelmingly. It was portrayed in the media as a victory for the elderly and a triumph of progressive taxation. In fact, it called for the elderly to bear the entire cost of the program by imposing a special surtax on all elderly persons paying $150 or more a year in income tax. In short, the bill was actually a means of transferring the social cost of catastrophic care from the rich to those less able to pay. When the elderly realized this, they reacted with anger and ultimately brought about the bill's repeal in 1989. Unfortunately, the media, relying on their own misrepresentations of what the bill was about, have portrayed the elderly as selfish people who do not want to pay their fair share.

Be nice to your kids Melinda Beck, *Newsweek* 115:72–3+ Mr 12 '90

Congress is facing the controversial issue of who should pay for long-term care for elderly patients. More than 6 million elderly Americans now need basic long-term care, and the number will grow in the coming decades as the nation's population ages and life expectancy increases. Recently, the U.S. Bipartisan Commission on Comprehensive Health Care issued a list of recommendations. The panel called for legislation to provide universal basic health care and for the creation of a giant social-insurance program to guarantee home care and nursing-home care to all severely disabled citizens who need these services. Critics, including many members of Congress, believe that such an approach would compound the anticipated exponential increase in Social Security and Medicare costs.

There's nothing universal about plans for universal health care Susan B. Garland, *Business Week* 39 Ja 22 '90

Most lawmakers, businessmen, labor leaders, insurers, and doctors agree that the time has come for a national health care policy but they cannot agree on what the policy should look like. Democratic senator John D. Rockefeller IV of West Virginia, who chairs the Bipartisan Commission on Comprehensive Health Care, believes that all employers should either provide benefits or pay a tax to fund a federal program for the uninsured. Many small companies oppose this plan, fearing that the costs would be overwhelming. Big corporations like the idea because they believe that small companies are indirectly responsible for rising medical costs. Doctors, state governments, insurers, and various special interest groups are worried about the effects of any plan on them. Lawmakers will probably not take any action on the issue until after the 1990 elections.

No more health care on the house (Fortune poll) Alan Farnham, *Fortune* 119:71–2 F 27 '89

The top CEOs in the United States view health care as an increasing burden. Health care now consumes more than 11 percent of the GNP, and businesses are paying 45 percent of operating profits to foot the nation's medical bill. According to the latest Fortune 500/CNN Moneyline CEO poll, present and retired employees are increasingly being asked to pick up at least part of the tab. More CEOs favor national health coverage than ever, although a large majority still opposes it.

National health care is fundamental for a great modern nation J. R. Joelson, *The Humanist* 50:35–6 Mr/Ap '90

Although nearly 12 percent of the U.S. gross national product is spent on health care, 15 percent of all Americans have no medical coverage. This situation contributes to unemployment and homelessness because people who have no medical insurance and who work in marginal situations could lose their jobs when illness strikes. The United States should follow the lead of its economic competitors and adopt a system of universal health care.

The right medicine Harry Schwartz, *National Review* 41:26–9 Mr 10 '89

The high cost of health care and the substantial number of Americans without health insurance have sparked a barrage of criticism of the health care system. The fact is that these two problems have arisen directly from policies that these same critics supported. For many years, the dominant political culture has been calling for an American health care system equivalent to those in Europe that allow free health care for everyone, regardless of income. This has been largely achieved, creating a boom in the health care field that has sparked a rise in prices. The problem could be solved by a plan that provides universal catastrophic illness insurance but otherwise makes the patient responsible for selecting and paying for health care.

Koop de grace *The New Republic* 201:7–9 O 23 '89

Former surgeon-general C. Everett Koop was an excellent adviser to the citizenry on matters of public health. After stirring up the populace about smoking, AIDS, and the importance of improved diet and regular exercise, he drew attention during his last summer in office to the sad state of the United States' system of health care. Without endorsing socialized medicine, Koop supports some form of national health provision, an idea that is gaining support outside liberal circles. A state-based version of the Canadian system that would be financed by excise taxes and a new payroll tax could work for the United States. To establish such a system, Congress would have to approve a tax increase and stand up to the powerful lobbies representing hospitals, insurers, and doctors. An endorsement from Koop would be an excellent way to launch the campaign for a comprehensive health care system.

Some of the tough decisions required by a national health plan
Louise B. Russell, *Science* 246:892–6 N 17 '89

The goals of providing coverage for everyone in the United States and controlling the growth in national health expenditures require difficult decisions about what medical services to provide. Currently accepted practices vary enormously in the amount of health they produce for a given expenditure. Studies of the health effects of several major interventions in relation to their costs—Pap smears, mammography, coronary care units, bypass surgery, and cholesterol reduction—indicate the kinds of choices to be made. Copyright 1989 by the AAAS.

Society, cure thyselfe Daniel E. Koshland, Jr., *Science* 248:9 Ap 6 '90

The time has come for the United States to devise a national health insurance system that is both equitable and affordable. Any good health care system will be expensive, but it could save money in the long run. Moreover, many steps could be taken to contain costs. For example, limits could be placed on malpractice suits, and people could be required to pay for especially costly or fancy procedures with their own money.

Lessons from Canada's health program Milton Terris, *Technology Review* 93:26–33 F/Mr '90

The United States has much to learn from the strengths and weaknesses of the Canadian health insurance system. Many Americans wish that their government would emulate aspects of the Canadian health system, such as universal coverage, payment in full, and funding through progressive taxes. Adopting such features would in fact ease the growing problem of inequitable health coverage in the United States. The Canadian plan, however, shares several of the American system's other shortcomings, like fee-for-service pricing, an inadequate emphasis on disease prevention, and a failure to monitor quality of care. Instead of copying the Canadian system, the United States should remove costs from the control of the medical profession by making annual payments to health provider organizations rather than to individual practitioners. In addition, it should double its annual expenditures on public health and develop federal standards for quality control.